All About
The Baby Sleep Solution

Your Questions Answered

Lucy Wolfe

Gill Books

Gill Books
Hume Avenue
Park West
Dublin 12
www.gillbooks.ie

Gill Books is an imprint of M.H. Gill and Co.

978 07171 8554 2

Designed by Síofra Murphy
Print origination by O'K Graphic Design, Dublin
Copy-edited by Emma Dunne
Proofread by Djinn von Noorden
Indexed by Cliff Murphy
Printed by CPI Group (UK) Ltd, Croydon CRO 4YY

This book is typeset in Adobe Caslon Pro and Slabo.

The paper used in this book comes from the wood pulp of managed forests.
For every tree felled, at least one tree is planted, thereby renewing natural
resources.

5 4 3 2 1

Acknowledgements

To my lovely husband Alan, who listens, makes suggestions and, more importantly, supports me. Nothing overwhelms you – you are a steady influence and constant supplier of chocolate whom I love and need. Without you I would not be where I am today. You underpin the whole foundation of our lovely life.

To my wonderful children Jesse, Ellen, Eden and Harry – every day is an adventure. I celebrate each one of you and I am in awe of your wisdom, confidence and growth into amazing people whom I get to call mine and spend all my time with. You ARE my favourite people; it's true.

To the team at Gill Books: Sarah Liddy, Catherine Gough, Teresa Daly, Paul Neilan, Mairead O'Keeffe and the rest of the team. Thank you – I appreciate all your support, guidance and patience.

Most of all, though, sincere thanks to all of the parents who invite me into their lives and allow me to be part of their sleep journeys, who trust and recommend me to others, and help spread the word, who discuss me, post about me, tag me, like my posts, comment, message me, DM me, buy my books, my products and engage my services. I never tire of hearing how sharing my craft has made a difference. I am always very emotional when I hear and see that helping you in any way has made your lives easier. It is a privilege. Parenting *is* hard, that is the truth – with better sleep and, more importantly, understanding, each age and stage becomes more manageable. I thank you for letting me be part of that with you.

Contents

Introduction

Hello, it's so lovely to meet you. I always consider it an honour and a privilege when families invite me into their lives to help improve their sleep. So first, let me say thank you for trusting in me and allowing me to be part of your journey.

After I wrote *The Baby Sleep Solution*, I didn't think I would ever write another book – I found it very hard to work and parent full-time *and* write. I was also apprehensive about what disclosing my work and methods in this way might do to my private practice.

I need not have worried. The way that parents have been helped, supported and reassured by *The Baby Sleep Solution* has meant so much to me – my private practice became even busier, my platform larger and my voice, much needed among the conflicting and sometimes inappropriate sleep advice out there for parents to pick through, heard.

Following a break from the pressures of writing, I felt there was scope to tackle issues parents were reporting surrounding their efforts, and that taking sleep in sections and replying to the common queries that arise would further help families keen to encourage their child to sleep better. My approach hasn't changed, but what you've told me has informed adjustments I have made and how I describe certain sleep elements.

I know that immediate results are desirable and, as a tired parent, having to read a whole book may not suit. So in this book, although you may still need to read quite a bit, you can select your problem area and link the chapters back and forth as you go.

Seventeen years ago, when I became a parent for the first time, there were no readily available internet or social media platforms. The existing approaches to helping children sleep better did not sit well with me, and I began a journey to become a support and advocate for a gentle parent-accompanied method that bridged the gap between cry-intensive approaches or never sleeping again.

As a mum of four children, I know first hand how different each child can be and how challenging parenting can be too. I hope this book helps to provide solutions, reassurance, confidence and empowerment for those of you looking for answers and seeking a holistic approach that prioritises your parenting philosophies and your child's emotional and developmental well-being, as well as establishing positive sleep practices that can last for all time.

Lucy Wolfe

Chapter 1

Your Baby's Sleep

Understanding sleep

Experiencing sleep challenges with your infant or child can have an extremely debilitating effect on the entire family unit. Everybody's situation and every child is different, thus not every suggestion or adjustment will work for you. But most changes suggested here will help move you further towards better sleep.

I don't expect children to 'sleep through the night' at an early age. This term is overused and not entirely understood. Typically, when it is age appropriate – from six months onwards – you can try to enable your child to sleep longer and deeper. This means more consolidated stretches of sleep with minimised parental input, ranging from necessary night feeds to comfort and reassurance. Basically, you try to establish the optimum level of sleep for your child (and you) at that moment in time and then continue to enhance, improve and future-proof this.

Not all sleep challenges require intervention – very often what you may be experiencing are typical childhood sleep patterns, especially in the first six months of life, together with routine disturbances for older children.

When your baby is born, they are immature in every sense – including their nervous system, their digestive system and, of course, their sleeping patterns. Young babies are designed to wake and feed frequently. While this can be draining and frustrating, it may be easier if we reframe our expectations and stop thinking that babies 'should' and 'must' be doing certain things by specific points in time.

Lucy Says

Having expectations set by outside influences only undermines our parenting experience and lowers our self-esteem and confidence in our treatment of our child and ourselves. I firmly believe that in the first six months of your child's life you should have low expectations – yes, it is hard, it is challenging and you may be more tired than you have ever been, but you can slowly begin to work behind the scenes to nudge your child's sleep into a more improved sleep space – always in the context of first ensuring that they feel loved, safe, responded to and secure.

Q So what is a sleep problem, then?

For me, a sleep problem that requires or would benefit from intervention is only applicable once your child is at least six months of age. Before then, although it can feel like a problem, changes you make may not have much effect. It is worth applying my early months sleep-shaping suggestions (see page 61), but it is not until six months and beyond, developmentally, that I feel a more intense approach is appropriate. And, at that, we will never try to impose better sleep at the emotional expense of your baby (or the rest of the family) – everything that we do needs to be meaningful, emotionally connected and entirely ring-fenced by loving responses.

I encourage parents to view their child's sleep in two parts: under six months, where we undertake sleep shaping; and six months and beyond, where we implement sleep learning as needed. The reasoning behind this partition is sleep maturation and ensuring that your baby is ready, developmentally and emotionally, for some of the adjustments that you may need to make to help them sleep better.

As a practitioner, I work directly with families with children from six months to six years of age. This is for several reasons:

- Before this age range there is a lot of variability, and although there are changes that you can make, it's not until at least six months – and later for others – that a sleep-learning exercise can have a positive impact.
- Although the tiredness that you experience can be debilitating and frustrating, as your child gets older, you can very much help them to become more robust sleepers – it is not just the way they are.
- Although I encourage you to wait and see what needs to be addressed, sometimes issues may not go away with time, solid food, movement or age, and it will be necessary to undertake some element of sleep work to reach your sleep goals for your family unit.
- It is never too late to begin a sleep improvement exercise, whatever your child's age. Each age range has its own set of challenges, and each temperament has its own trials, but you have never missed the opportunity: you can begin today.

I cap my one-to-one work at six years of age because I work directly with the *parents* rather than the child. Although many of my treatments can be successfully applied to children older than six, they may benefit from working directly with a mentor or therapist too, as the emotional landscape shifts with age and many social elements come into play that might be best addressed with that child being accompanied by a professional.

Q What common sleep challenges do parents report?

Common sleep challenges are often represented by some of the following tendencies:

- You find it difficult to get your child to go to sleep at bedtime.
- Your child finds it hard to maintain their sleep overnight – they may wake frequently, anything from every 45 minutes to every 2–4 hours.

- They stay awake for long period of time overnight – from 1 to 3–5 hours.
- They wake early – from 4–5 a.m. onwards – either having woken a lot during the night or slept until this time.
- You have no difficulty getting your child to sleep but they still find it hard to stay asleep through the night.
- They will only go back to sleep with milk or water feeds.
- They will only allow a certain parent to help them sleep.
- They resist daytime sleep.
- They fail to achieve close to their suggested daytime sleep needs – only staying asleep for 20–40 minutes at a time.
- You spend a lot of your day trying to get them to sleep, only to have a small burst of sleep in return.
- You spend 1–3 hours trying to get them asleep at bedtime and they do stay asleep once this heroic effort has been applied.

Parents can report any one of the above, a combination or a rolling cycle of some days better or worse, some nights better or worse or a tag team between the issues over the course of days, weeks or months.

If you are experiencing any or all of the above with your six-month or older child, for at least a month (so we know that teething, sickness or a developmental leap is not the cause) *and* we can rule out any underlying medical issues, then you have a sleep challenge that can be addressed and, of course, more importantly, improved on.

UNDERLYING MEDICAL ISSUES

A vast array of underlying medical issues could undermine your child's sleep, and it is important to rule out the possibility that something medical is a barrier. But it is equally important to ensure you are not blaming something that is only part of what you are experiencing. Once any medical issue is identified and controlled/managed then sleep can, in turn, be enhanced.

The most common medical issues are digestive problems – food sensitivities, intolerances and reflux can certainly make it hard to sleep

– but once these are diagnosed and managed correctly then, despite having what I call a 'reflux hangover', derived from what you have done to meet this need in the early months, great sleep can be expected too. Even if you are unsure whether the condition is controlled, making the changes I suggest will help you establish what is causing what.

I have worked with many children with various diagnoses – cerebral palsy, severe brain trauma, ADHD and autism, to name but a few – and although we see some variability, it is not enormous, so the message is really that everyone can be helped to sleep longer, deeper and better.

Also, even with a diagnosis of any kind, I don't make any specific adjustments to the plan unless you, as parent, feel sure a certain recommendation would not suit your child and then we can modify accordingly.

Q Who can have a sleep problem?

The answer is anyone! It doesn't matter who you are, what you do for a living, how many children you have had, how well read or prepared you may be, sleep challenges can happen to anyone.

And it does not mean you have done something wrong. Many parents feel that their child's sleeping (or lack of it) is their fault, that they have failed and that they 'should' be able to help their child sleep. I see this very differently and hope to reassure you that there is no right or wrong way. Certainly, some approaches work better than others; but what worked for one child may not work for another and this does not mean anything: you have not failed; it is 'not all your own fault'; you have not 'made a rod for your own back'; it is not because you breastfed or didn't; gave a dummy or didn't; went back to work or decided to stay at home; or any other objection you might make.

Lucy Says

There is no right way or wrong way, but what there is is opportunity – embrace that. There are things you can do, there are changes you can make, and there is scope.

It is not 'just the way it is'; this is not 'just a parenting fact of life';

you do not have to accept multiple night-time awakenings – we can respectfully and gently enhance your child's sleep without compromising your parenting philosophies, giving up breastfeeding, ditching the soother, moving them into another room or putting them on eBay … Help is at hand!

You are already the expert, you just need to believe in yourself, your child and have faith in the plans and changes that I suggest. Trust your internal authority and stop second-guessing your choices. With my guidance you will all move into this more plentiful sleep land that I keep mentioning.

Q *Why do sleep problems happen?*

You may indeed say, why? Why do parents with a typically developing and healthy child seem to struggle so extensively with their sleep? How can it be that one parent who has prioritised their family sleep does not see a yield and another who is winging it gets a full night's sleep? How is that twins – who are eating and drinking the same – still differ so vastly in their sleep tendencies? Why does what you did with your first child not work for your second? Why, why, why?

Well, first, although I suggest sleep is straightforward, there are *so many* factors that affect your child's sleep:

- Everything *they* think, feel, see, do, hear, wear and eat drink affects their sleep.
- Everything *you* think, feel, see, do, hear, wear, eat and drink also affects *their* sleep.
- Everything the *other parent* thinks, feels and so on …

That is a lot of potential contributory factors to your child's sleeping ability!

Emotional wellbeing

In recent years, we've been hearing a lot about self-care, but I feel those words can get tossed around a bit. Self-care can be taking a break, going for a walk, having a mindful minute, but for me it is *so* much more than that. I place a lot of emphasis on your child's well-being and their emotional connectivity with you, helping them feel safe, secure and, in time, willing to be more separate from you – in life in general but in sleep specifically – when you are both ready.

Developmentally, your child will go through many milestones where they have attachment to the primary caregiver and then, in time, display some separation anxieties as they gain a greater sense of self. As parents, we acknowledge and accompany them through this as best we can.

What we also need to acknowledge is *our* emotional connection and availability within our own selves. It's important that we can first have a deep and meaningful relationship with ourselves, in an effort to establish the same with our children. Each one of us carries the traits, thoughts, expectations and anticipations established in our early years and getting beyond some or all of those will enable us as parents to speak and act from an authentic place and space.

Being kind, compassionate and patient with yourself, stopping the blaming or listening to the internal critic that may be the soundtrack to your life, can start today. Coming from a loving place for yourself will radiate into the parent–child relationship and create beautiful opportunities for connection on every level.

This takes time and is, like improving sleep, an ongoing process. Understanding why you feel a certain way may help to diminish that feeling's power over you and start healing, one day at a time.

We know that *everything* can potentially affect your child's sleep, but there are two major contributory factors that have an overriding impact on child sleep tendencies:

1. Sleep ability
2. Timekeeping

Sleep ability

Anything you do to help your child get to sleep or back to sleep can potentially be an association that undermines your child's ability to stay asleep through their natural sleep phases.

There is absolutely nothing wrong with holding, feeding, rolling, rocking or lying down with your child to help them to go to sleep, *but*, unfortunately, the way that sleep is designed – and this kicks in at about 16 weeks, when sleep starts to mature and your child begins adult-like sleep phases – when you are involved *in any capacity* in helping them get to sleep, then you *may* be more vulnerable to unnecessary night-time activity that exceeds required feeds or comfort or reassurance tendencies.

Whatever you do with and for your baby or child as they're going to sleep, the brain may continually search for as it cycles through sleep phases. For example, you may use a bottle or breastfeed very close to bedtime or cuddle your baby all the way to sleep and transfer them to their cot relatively easily, and then within the first two to four hours they may call on you to do the same – or another association, such as walking about, feeding or bed-sharing – to help them back into their next sleep phase continually until morning time. As the night unfolds, the awakenings may become more frequent or prolonged and what worked earlier may be less helpful as the morning approaches so you need to change what you do. Then you may find that your child gets to about 5 a.m. and will either be alert and ready to start the day or go into another deep phase of sleep for an hour or more until morning time proper.

Whatever your child associates with going to sleep at bedtime can actually prevent them from staying asleep, as the brain and body search for continued help. Their sleep ability is incomplete. If you help in some capacity at bedtime, the exposure to unnecessary night-time waking is often exponentially increased.

Some parents feel there are no associations at bedtime, but continued dependency overnight. This may be the result of a hidden association or just that each time you attended to your baby in a certain way overnight has created expectations and further associations and so the waking continues.

Lucy Says

Although it can be hard to imagine, encouraging your child to achieve sleep at bedtime wholly for themselves and with less parental input without leaving them to cry alone will initiate the growth of an inherent ability to go to sleep with greater ease, and, perhaps more importantly, stay asleep for longer with more consolidated stretches. We will create complete sleep ability.

Remember, we are not necessarily expecting your child to 'sleep through' the night, but we are attempting to enable them to do so, if they are developmentally able, in a gentle and considerate way.

Timekeeping

This makes up 60–70 per cent of the issues reported. Briefly, it is all do with your child's circadian rhythm – their internal body clock. And guess what? It's not mature: it won't be until your child is perhaps four years. But it is extremely relevant from birth in how your child responds to their sleep.

Biological timekeeping comes down to what time your child wakes, what time you attempt their naps, how long they nap for, the gap between naps and when you start bedtime.

Children (and their parents) who struggle with sleep typically have irregular (too early or too late) wake times. Their daytime sleep is often attempted when already overtired and as a result the naps are varied – too short or too long in duration – the balance between the sleeps is out of sync and the bedtime is addressed when your child is overtired or out of balance with their natural rhythm, and it is *this* that largely contributes to the following sleep issues:

- Resisting sleep
- Unable to maintain sleep – waking frequently

- Waking within an hour of bedtime
- Staying awake for long periods
- Early rising
- Short naps

It is a vicious cycle and almost self-fulfilling prophecy. Overtiredness breeds overtiredness: your child wakes overnight, they start the day overtired (despite your best efforts), they are too tired to take a nap or they nap for too long – the balance now between sleeps is too long or too short and the nap-gap dynamic (see page 174) is creating an *imbalance* that means your child goes to sleep too early or too late, they wake and the cycle continues, digging both of you into a deeper hole of sleep deprivation, right?

It's all so overwhelming – what can we do?

- Up to six months – gentle sleep shaping (outlined in Chapter 5)
- Six months to six years – gentle sleep learning

We attempt to strengthen timekeeping by applying the feeding and sleeping balances in Chapters 6 and 9 (my first book, *The Baby Sleep Solution*, goes into further detail, so you can refer back to it if you need more information). The age-appropriate feeding and sleeping suggestions aim to 'hijack' your child's biological rhythm and help create a balance between feeds and sleeps.

Do your best to follow *all* of the guidelines, as experience has shown me that the 'sleep deal is in the sleep detail' and can make the difference between things staying the same (or getting worse) and starting to *feel* different and improving.

Lucy Says

When we begin the sleep-learning exercises and as we strengthen the timekeeping as outlined, we will start to enhance sleep ability. To do this, we will use my stay-and-support approach to transition from what you currently do to help your child fall asleep and stay asleep. This is outlined in Chapter 3, along with the stages to sleep, and I will refer to both regularly as I address the common questions that arise.

Chapter 2
Barriers to Sleep Success

The changes I will encourage you to make are both evidence *and* practice based, formed through my work over the years and continually refined while assisting parents through their challenging and frustrating sleep issues. My aim in this book is to widen my one-to-one consultation work, but sometimes the only remedy is to work directly with a practitioner to receive a personalised individual plan with support and guidance to reach your goals. Don't be afraid to reach out if you feel that the journey on your own is too overwhelming, because it can happen. But that said, literally thousands of parents have mastered great sleep by applying my strategies and suggestions from *The Baby Sleep Solution*.

A number of factors can reduce the chances of your sleep-learning plan working, and I want to outline them for you so that all your efforts will give a yield and help you to reach your goals – provided they are realistic in the first place.

Lucy Says

Realistic for me is understanding that children do wake; they do require parental input and depend on you; they are entitled to night-time feeds – sometimes for longer than you would like; and they will probably wake earlier than adults like too. They generally won't sleep later on the weekend; they probably won't sleep in if you put them to bed later. They probably will wake a lot if they are sick or teething; they may just like to see you overnight if they have not connected with you much that day. But they can be encouraged to sleep more, to need less input, to eat better and to demonstrate enhanced mood and behaviour when they are optimally rested.

'Understanding my little boy's sleep has taken so much anxiety away from nap and bedtime.'

— Sarah, mum to six-month-old Max

I often hear of parents who have 'tried everything', whether from a book – mine or another's – through forums, advice online, tips from friends and relatives, yet they really feel that their child 'just won't sleep'. Beyond six months, there are some main factors that, together or separately, can dilute your efforts:

1. Bedtime addressed too late or when the child is already overtired

2. Nap imbalance or nap-deprivation dynamic

3. Reduced level of sleep ability

4. Overnight not yet addressed consistently

We'll look at each of these points in detail below.

1. Late bedtimes

Generally, an early onset of sleep helps your child go to sleep with greater ease and stay asleep for longer. Bedtime for young children, from about four months to six-years-plus ranges between 6 and 8 p.m. However, when your child is not routinely sleeping well, then nothing is early enough! Even 7.15 p.m. or 7.30 p.m. is too late when your child does not usually sleep well overnight and/or by day too.

Perhaps your child's night-time sleep *is* good but daytime sleep *isn't*. When bedtime is slightly too late biologically, it can prevent daytime sleep happening with ease, so observing an earlier bedtime tends to support better sleep overall – both overnight and by day.

To further help you, I have devised the bedtime number line (see page 133) to encourage you to practise an earlier bedtime when age appropriate and when hoping to achieve increased sleep by day and by night. This will help you stop attempting bedtime too late.

Q *I'm worried that an earlier bedtime will mean that he will be awake even earlier!*

When I mention early bedtimes in group settings, parents often have objections – 'it seems too early', 'I'm worried about the wake time in the morning', 'I won't see my child – I'm barely home from work then' – and I understand those concerns. But if you really want to improve your child's sleep and promote longer sleeping durations then observing an early (in bed asleep by 7 p.m.) bedtime is a necessary adjustment in most instances.

Once you have improved your child's sleep then it may be possible to push bedtime back out again, or indeed, if despite starting early your child never achieves sleep until a certain later time, then there is scope to start later and not be under as much pressure.

However, for those of you whose children fall asleep very close to 7 p.m., that represents their natural bedtime. Moving it later may undermine your previous efforts and night waking and early rising may re-emerge unless the early bedtime is continually observed. This is about meeting a need – your child's need to sleep by a certain time, resulting in a happier, more rested individual.

2. Nap deprivation

Achieving enough daytime sleep for your child can have immediate positive implications for night-time sleep. There is a distinct relationship between the quality of the daytime sleep and the deepness of the night-time sleep. If your child does not get enough daytime sleep then you may be exposed to unwanted night-time activity, as an overtired child will be more inclined to wake and require parental support to return to sleep.

Q How much sleep should my child be getting at nine months?

I try not to have parents count the hours of sleep, as I believe that if we create the right dynamic the body will respond in kind. Don't forget, your child's body is designed to sleep – mostly we just need to program them correctly, and once we start to achieve sleep at the right time, then the body can stay asleep for as long as it needs to, thus eliminating the negative overtired cycle (with some adjustments, of course).

That said, there are general nap-amount recommendations (see Chapter 14), and if your child does not get enough day sleep or significantly less than proposed, then you are going to be more vulnerable to night-time activity. Only use this as a guide, though, not to fill a quota per se.

BALANCING NAPS

My main focus with naps is the balance between sleeps. The age-appropriate feeding and sleeping balances up to eighteen months that I suggest (see page 95) describe the wake-window timing within which to attempt to help your child to sleep. Once we observe a smaller wake period between waking in the morning and first and second naps, when applicable, then we are starting to create the correct balance for sleep, and your child will typically go to sleep easier and sleep longer, thereby achieving their optimum need for sleep. This is then replaced with clock-based timings (see page 108) – all of the adjustments are to ensure that the vulnerabilities to sleep issues are continually reducing.

NAP-GAP DYNAMIC

A number of nap tendencies can diminish your efforts for better sleep – one in particular is the wake period between the final nap end and being in bed asleep. My nap-gap dynamic honours the relationship between naps and bedtime and the science of sleep and in doing so helps to unlock your child's sleep ability.

The nap-gap dynamic observes an age-relevant wake period between daytime and night-time sleep, without which we tend to see unnecessary waking overnight and a variety of other issues.

Some families may try to finish the naps later and still observe the suggested nap-gap dynamic together with a later bed timing, and this can sometimes work, but as it may challenge the internal body clock, it can prove less effective. My general recommendation is to start on my timeline and adjust when the sleep has been improved and you have a 'working model'.

Even with precise timing, if you do not adequately prepare your child for sleep, you often see a high level of objection come bedtime. This is where you can utilise the power of the bedtime routine. While we rely heavily on melatonin hormonal secretion and sleep pressure to help with bedtime, a pre-sleep ritual will further augment the message that it is time to sleep.

🇶 *My baby gets enough sleep as per their age range but I still don't see better sleep overnight.*

Another nap imbalance is when your child is getting enough sleep on paper, but if they are still on more than one nap we often see:

- **Naps power play:** The first nap overpowers the day, resulting in a weaker second nap and, as a result, still being overtired at bedtime. Clipping the naps as outlined in my sleeping and feeding suggestions will ensure we are balancing naps for the day.

- **Naps over too early:** When toddlers transition to one nap, I frequently see the nap happening too early in the day, and although bedtime is at the appropriate time, the wake-time gap far exceeds the four to five hours they can tolerate before becoming so overtired that they crash or battle at bedtime, leaving you further exposed to long wake periods and early rising (we'll explore this further in Chapter 14).

3. Sleep ability

As mentioned in Chapter 1, sleep ability exists on a spectrum:

- Low sleep ability – requires parent to help them go entirely to sleep
- Incomplete sleep ability – requires a level of input, sometimes not obvious: possibly a feed too close to sleep time or a parent's presence or input as they go asleep
- Complete sleep ability – can put themselves to sleep without a parent present or a feed too close to sleep time

So if you routinely feed or rock or lie with your child until they are asleep, or transfer them from arms to cot or bed to cot pretty much asleep, then you tick the low sleep ability box. And while many families do this and their child sleeps through the night, countless others find their child is waking too many times to mention, or their day sleep is compromised even if the night is manageable.

If after adjusting the timings and laying a foundation of night-time sleep it still feels unmanageable, then your child may need to learn how to be more sleep 'able' – to develop their *own* ability to fall asleep and cycle through at least some of their sleep phases without parental input.

My stay-and-support approach (see page 26) enables you to transition from low to complete sleep ability without the need to allow your child to cry unattended. Although there may well be crying, it is parent attended and child led, and bolstered by all the foundations that support emotional wellbeing together with better sleep.

Q *I feel that I do everything you suggest, yet I'm not making the progress I anticipated*

In my private practice, one of the most diluting factors I find is the incomplete sleep ability, or what I have previously described as a *partial dependency* – one that is not obvious – where parents report that their child is independent or 'sleep able' at bedtime, but the sleep issues overnight remain. An incomplete sleep ability happens normally when the final feed – although separate to bedtime or not the last thing that you do – is still too close to sleep time. I find that, unless there is a definite 45 minutes between the end of the feed and the time you are aiming for your child to be asleep, it is still potentially too close. That final act of sucking on the breast, bottle or cup is enabling a sleepy state, making going asleep easy but disabling the ability to maintain sleep overnight as a result. To remedy this, I have introduced my fixed-feed concept, which you can align with all the other suggestions. It may also be that you are still present as they go to sleep, barely doing anything, but without your being there, they may not go to sleep with such ease, leaving you more exposed to unnecessary night-time activity.

Lucy Says

If your child goes into their sleep space on a final feed and sleeps through and naps well, no action is required. If the opposite is true, I would encourage further adjustments to ensure that your child really is putting themselves entirely to sleep at bedtime and, as a result, is more competent at cycling through night-sleep phases.

Even if you make this change tonight, the night waking will remain until it too is treated, as expectation and association on your child's part will be deeply ingrained. That is where your patience and commitment to change and improvement are required as part of the plan.

THE FIXED FEED

From six months onwards, I encourage the concept of the fixed feed, which means that the final milk feed is *finished* at least 45 minutes to 1 hour before bedtime. Although *The Baby Sleep Solution* has helped many families, I still meet parents who either misinterpret this message or do not see its relevance or importance. It is a very important adjustment and can make all the difference to your progress.

Q *My child refuses to drink the fixed feed*

I often hear that a child won't drink their bottle unless they're in the bedroom, or they will only breastfeed without distractions in a dark room. And of course, I hear that parents are worried about hunger and that having a feed directly before bedtime is supposed to keep children asleep – whereas I can honestly say the opposite is true. Although sucking is relaxing and breast milk has the right properties to induce sleep, if sucking close to sleep time is your child's association with achieving sleep then this may need to be repeated potentially many times through the night because sleep has its own designs. This is addressed with my bedtime number line (see page 133) and by routinely removing the final feed, whether it's finished or not, by 6.15 p.m.

4. Overnight not addressed consistently

This barrier occurs when you have made all the suggested daytime and bedtime changes but you have not yet completely addressed the night-time waking. In the following chapters, you will see that sleep exists in segments and each segment requires intervention to adequately address your challenges. This means you will require a plan to help diminish the expectation of the approaches you have historically taken overnight. For some of you, this will include night weaning or regulating night feeds and erasing a cycle of waking to be fed, bed-sharing, starting the day too soon or any other strategy that you invoke to get your child back to sleep – iPads, phones, TV, water, feeds: the list is endless.

Many of you will apply the plan overnight and still report no improvement. This generally indicates that something by day and possibly at bedtime is not adequately aligned or has been misinterpreted. Some of you will just have to work on the overnight and sleep segments, acknowledging that this often takes the longest to address and is, to be fair, the hardest, as this is when we ourselves would like to be in bed sleeping.

Lucy Says

Consider this time spent overnight addressing expectations and growing sleep ability as an investment in your child's sleep in perpetuity, so the yield of your effort will pay dividends for this hard and challenging project.

These are the main diluting factors, and the following chapters will provide deeper context and answer the questions that recur for those parents who are struggling. Hopefully, we are gaining understanding and confidence in making changes that will allow some great things to start to happen!

> *'I bought your book out of sheer desperation and what a difference it has made. It has been a week now and there have been zero feeds at night. Two naps during the day and up to bed at 7 p.m. and sleeping until 7.15 a.m. Granted he wakes once or so just for a bit of a cuddle and back down again – I mean, literally two minutes and he falls back asleep when I put him in. With stay-and-support there are still tears but it's to be expected! I followed everything except the last feed before bedtime a few weeks back and it didn't work … as soon as I gave the last feed 45 minutes before bed it changed everything, so thank you a thousand times over. You are a life saver.'*
> *– Aide, mum to seven-month-old Gemma*

Chapter 3

Growing Your Sleep

When we attempt to improve any child's sleep – I call this 'growing your sleep' – it is best to start from ground level and work upwards. Parents will get a much better result when an entirely holistic approach is applied.

Many times, due to external pressure, families immediately starting applying a sleep-training technique like controlled crying, cry it out or, indeed, a gradual retreat like my stay-and-support approach, without first addressing the backstory. Treatments that do not fully encompass every aspect of your child's health and development can often result in unnecessary upset and distress for parent and child. It can mean night upon night of endless tears that don't even produce the desired effect.

Lucy Says

In my experience, the backstory – your child's age and stage, the feeding and sleeping balance, the timing, the preparation, the environment and the emotional setting – may not be established enough, and this dilutes your efforts and leads you to think you will never sleep again. Not true! But you need to walk before you try to run.

Setting the context

As discussed in the previous chapters, multiple factors affect your child's sleep – where they sleep, what they sleep in, how they feed, exercise, fresh air and so on. To give yourself the best chance of success, the following basics should be addressed before applying my or any other sleep solution:

- Environment should be sleep inducing: blackout blind, curtains, avoid hall lights and bathroom light – use a night light (very dim) plugged into the wall, not the ceiling. Remove distractions such as cot toys with the exception of a security item, such as a safe breathable blanket that your baby can hold and associate with sleep time.
- Remove sleep positioners, bumpers, mobiles and excess bedding.
- Be mindful of the safe sleep guidelines (see appendix, p. 212).
- Ensure they are warm enough – recommended 16–20°c – and dressed for the season. Ideally, use a sleeping bag until they're ready to transition to a big bed. There are lots of options out there – ones with feet, without feet, arms, zips, Velcro – find what works for you and adjust to the season.
- Ensure they've had enough to eat and drink per age and stage – continually review.
- Engage in plenty of outside activity and fresh air – one hour a day (more if you like) is the recommendation: aim for 30 minutes in the morning and again in the afternoon. For older children, ensure that it is high-level activity – playing in the garden, park or playground or cycling or scooting, for example – and that you balance being sedentary with action.
- Avoid screen time, especially within an hour of bedtime, and as best as possible (not at all if you can) by day.
- Note that if we make changes, we always do so at bedtime, and the day you begin, follow the suggested feeding and sleep balance for your child's age range as precisely as possible but

continue to achieve sleep as you have been – rocking, feeding, bed-sharing – whatever works.

- Ensure that you are spending good quality time with your child – plenty of floor time, eye contact and physical and verbal communication.
- Using my stay-and-support approach to improve sleep ability before six months is not recommended – until then follow all my suggestions for under six months and then review. Using the approach before your child is developmentally ready can make everything more challenging and also not give you the desired results.
- Using my feeding and sleeping balances as closely as you can at the start makes the whole process work easier, so try your best to follow the framework.
- Make sure you have at least a three- to four-week window to devote to enhancing your child's sleep – avoid weekends away, sleepovers and major disruptions outside of unplanned events such as teething and sickness.
- Don't have any vaccinations during the timeframe and start when at least five days have passed since the most recent injections, sickness or teething period has elapsed.

EXPECTED OUTCOMES

Ideally, once you are following my suggestions your child will start to be able to achieve and maintain their sleep with minimised parental input – acknowledging that your child may always need support, comfort and reassurance from you in some capacity, both at bedtime and overnight, together with whatever necessary feeds they require, based on age, stage and personal preferences. Improvements take time to emerge, so ring-fence a month or more, within which time your child's sleep can be established.

We aim to optimally consolidate your child's night-time sleep and anticipate a wake time of not before 6 a.m., and ideally later – though this is not always achievable. What you will establish, though, is your child's natural sleep tendency.

Your child may also be able to take age-relevant daytime sleep – in a cot, bed or wherever you have decided. This daytime sleep, along with night-time sleep and feeding, will be synchronised with my suggested dynamics to support and futureproof your child's sleep.

In this chapter you will see how I help a child transition from low or incomplete sleep ability at bedtime and overnight and how this will help later on. Ensure, however, that you work through *all* the stages – or as much as your child will accept. Regardless of the challenges, big or small, this is a process, and once you begin to expose the contributory factors, you then need to continue to make changes quite rapidly to ensure that your sleep goals are achieved.

It may sometimes get worse before it gets better – your typical smooth bedtime may unravel, night waking may become more frequent, longer and more tiring, but that is often the nature of the 'undoing', as I call it.

Whatever changes you make will cause a shift – removing a feed that was too close to sleep time may mean that you need to support your child when you would normally leave the room – but this is actually positive. A struggle at bedtime, supported by you, means that the feed *was* enabling falling asleep, but in turn disabling staying asleep. This struggle will resolve quite quickly, and although the night waking and early rising may continue, if you continue methodically, respectfully and meaningfully then you will start to see a yield within a four-week timeframe. Acknowledge that it takes time, patience and commitment to grow their sleep tendency.

If your child is upset when you make the transition to my method then use my stay-and-support approach to replace anything that you would have done historically. If they are calm at bedtime and do not need comfort then leave as normal and only use as required.

The stay-and-support approach

This is a sleep-learning alternative to controlled crying, cry it out, pick-up put-down, shush-pat or any other cry-intensive sleep 'training' technique.

As a parent and practitioner, I never want your or my child to be upset, but realistically I know that if you are transitioning them from

certain sleep associations that do not seem to support their night-
or daytime sleep, then there may be protest, upset or distress as they
process the changes you are making.

You may never have to use a strategy like this if you observe the
sleep-shaping suggestions and/or make the timing adjustments and,
through those changes alone, your child's sleep emerges naturally or
improves. But if you find that those changes alone have not moved
the needle in the right direction, then encouraging greater sleep ability
may become necessary.

When this is the case, that transition should be parent-attended,
supported by you – emotionally, physically and developmentally – so
the end result (better sleep) is never a compromise or at the expense
of your child's emotional wellbeing, but an acknowledgement that
changes are necessary for improvement, and that, for your child to
accept those changes, they need your guidance and support. As they
manage and discover a slightly different way of going or staying asleep,
they need you to accompany them, to hold them emotionally, on their
pathway to sleep ability.

Lucy Says

If something instinctively doesn't feel right for you – deep in your gut
– then it's not for you. If it resonates with you, reassures you, gives you
confidence and motivation, if your child, despite initially being upset,
takes on the changes, if it starts to feel different, better, stronger and at
all times appropriate for your family, then I hope you will continue and
that better sleep is coming your way.

Stay-and-support should be used as required having observed the
feeding and sleeping balance for your child's age (six months plus)
and first making the changes, if applicable, at bedtime. If your child is
calm then you don't need to stay, but if they are not calm and
need support – which is to be expected – then use the method as
detailed here.

Position yourself on the floor (use a chair only if your child is still in the high level of a cot), down at your child's level, beside the cot, where you can easily comfort, reassure and support your child as they learn the process of sleep. Make yourself comfortable – you may be a while – and stay patient and calm: it takes time to learn something new. It is progressive learning on your child's part.

The elements of stay-and-support are:

1. Physically respond

2. Verbally respond

3. Use distraction

4. Manage sitting or standing up

5. Pick up to calm

6. Stay until fast asleep

We'll look at each of these in detail below.

1. PHYSICALLY RESPOND

You can comfort your child physically with stroking, rubbing and patting through and over the bars of the cot. Touching your child will let them know that you are there and help to regulate their autonomic nervous system. What does your child like?

- Stroking the temples
- Stroking the bridge of the nose
- Rubbing the back of the neck
- Doing a pat-pat-shush on their side or torso
- Walking your fingers up their body
- Swirling your hands over their tummy
- Doing a tom-tom rhythm on their body
- Rolling them on their side
- Wiggling their torso

Some of these responses may seem too interactive, but they can help support your child on this journey. Do these actions intermittently, as you're trying to avoid creating a new sleep association, but, at the same time, balance it with where you are coming from. This level of input helps to support your child as you transition them from an activity, such as feeding or rocking in arms, that does not support their ability long term, replacing it with this approach temporarily instead.

Try to ensure that you, the parent, are in charge of the touching. Avoid allowing your child to fall asleep holding your hand or finger. If they grab you, pat or rub a different part of the body, or tuck their hand in with their security item. If you *remain* hand-holding at sleep time, you may wake your child as you try to leave and ingrain a hyper-vigilance around falling asleep. You may also have to start the settling techniques all over again.

Lucy Says

If part of your child's expectations at bedtime or overnight involve hand-holding, then try to stop completely from night one onwards or use a security item between your hand and theirs. Concentrating on a different part of their body will help their transition – you'll be surprised how quickly they will adjust.

2. VERBALLY RESPOND

You can verbally reassure your child with shushing, humming, singing or using the broken-record technique – repeating the same sentence over and over (for example, 'It's sleep time, night-night'). You should maintain eye contact – even if the room is dark, as described earlier, and they cannot really see you, be there emotionally. Focus on their face. Letting your child know that you are there will keep their stress levels low during times of upset. Looking at them can help them to process the change with your considered responses.

🔲 *I don't think my child finds these strategies helpful*

I am the first to agree that these first two strategies can appear unhelpful. If your child is upset and crying, then touching may irritate them and they will swat you away, not wanting you near them. Have respect for that and reduce the touching. They also may not hear you if they are super-upset, so in that case, I would use my most effective settling tactic for settling: distraction.

3. USE DISTRACTION

Crying and sleep are not related. Your child does not need to cry to go to sleep. The crying is representative of the changes that you have made. It is typically a protest cry that cycles up and down. Your job is to bring the crying down, into quiet, so your child can start to fall asleep. This can sometimes happen rapidly, where your child is very upset one moment and then asleep the next. I recommend distraction to help manage the crying wave and give your child moments of pause and calm. Although the cry-free moments may not last long, and your child may start crying again, the pockets of calm can make your physical responses more effective. To distract, you can:

- Gently blow on their face
- Bang the bars of the cot
- Drum on the mattress
- Use white noise turned up loudly, then gradually turned down until off – unless you plan to use it all night
- Gently pat their chest to change the vibration of the crying
- Clap your hands
- Click your fingers

Lucy Says

If you gently blow on your child's face, you will stop them in their tracks – they may suck in their breath and in doing so present a moment of calm within which the stroking and rubbing can work more effectively, as they can concentrate on the touch. They will likely start up again, but you are being actively instrumental in helping them manage their level of upset.

Each distraction technique does not necessarily stop crying but they do help to manage the waves. You are being responsive and effective and supportive. Many parents report that they would never think of this strategy, as it doesn't necessarily fit with going to sleep, but keep in mind your child is not going to fall asleep crying: they need to self-regulate first and this can help.

4. MANAGE SITTING OR STANDING UP

Many children beyond the age of nine months will be able to stand or pull themselves up, and dealing with this can be a barrier to getting them to go to sleep. Teach your child how to be in the cot by staying down low on the floor beside them. However, if standing is a problem, then don't become involved in a power struggle – no one wins and very few children go to sleep on that basis. During the day:

- Practise going from standing to sitting to lying down with your child.
- Use key phrases like 'lie down', 'all fall down'.
- Playing ring-a-rosie can help.
- In the cot during non-sleep time, show them how to run their hands down the bars to sit.

If they stand at bedtime, naptime or overnight:

- First allow them to get it out of their system: let them do a lap of honour of the cot, then hug or comfort them and put them down *once* and return to your low position.
- If your child stands again, encourage them to come down on their own. Pat the mattress and stay low on the floor yourself.
- Don't get into a power struggle.
- Wait for your child to come down themselves using your key phrases.
- Your child may get sleepy or dozy at the cot-side while still standing – you can also lie them down then.

Can I pick them up? It's the million-dollar question and one every parent wants to know the answer to – most assuming it will be no. But …

5. PICK UP TO CALM

Of course you can pick them up to help them calm! I am not suggesting a pick-up put-down approach, as I feel it is too stimulating and unfair, especially if holding or rocking is your child's expectation, but I will always endorse a pick-up to prevent an indefinite cycle of crying. I would never want your child upset for an open-ended period of time, but I would also be conservative about picking up. Your child should come into a level of calm within 20–30 minutes of becoming upset. If possible, avoid picking them up within this time frame. If you feel you must pick them up, then absolutely do, but the more you pick up the longer it can take. If your child is hysterical, pick up and hold them until they're calmer, but don't allow them to fall asleep in your arms.

- Lift your child and shoulder cuddle/hold/rub/blow/comfort.
- Don't walk around or away from the cot.
- Once they take two to three calm breaths, return them to the cot.
- Resume your position and begin the settling techniques again.
- Often the child can become more upset on return – avoid lifting them immediately, as you will perpetuate the cycle. Instead begin again to apply the first few strategies and wait for the recommended 20–30 minutes.
- Decide if picking up helps – if it seems to only make your child worse, then it may suit better to be very conservative and use the first few strategies more intensively.

Lucy Says

It may be helpful to think of the approach as rungs of a ladder: go quickly up and down the physical, verbal and distraction steps, hold back on the pick-up step, and repeat as often as is required.

---

6. STAY UNTIL FAST ASLEEP

Don't leave the cot-side until your child is fast asleep and breathing regularly – normally after ten minutes it is safe. Do this at bedtime and during all night awakenings. Leaving too soon can waken them and make them hyper-vigilant.

Q *My child is rolling all about the cot and I keep stopping him – should I?*

If your child is rolling around the cot, allow them to do so – resist the urge to micromanage, rearrange or position them in a way that you feel is appropriate. Allow them to find what feels good for them. If they keep sitting up, treat this the same as standing up in the cot. Some children like to fall asleep sitting up and then all you need to do is gently lay them down once you feel they are sleepy enough.

Remember, you are creating space – physically and emotionally – for your child to go to sleep. If they are calm, you might want to attempt leaving, but they may only *be* calm because you are present. It's more effective to commit to the plan and the process.

It is highly possible that being present will overstimulate your child, but the only alternative is to leave and that is too intense at the start, although you can review and revert to the interval visits outlined on page 41 if you feel it might work. But, in the initial stages, staying and supporting is much more appropriate to help your child learn.

Stages to sleep

You have started a sleep-learning process, and there are stages you will need to go through to reach your end goals. We have set the scene, but we can't stay beside the cot forever, as this may start to become another challenge.

Q *We haven't moved through the stages that you outline*

I often meet families stuck in a first phase of sleep learning. They are beside the cot implementing a stay-and-support or a shush-pat approach or the widely used pick-up put-down strategy – they are stuck there and very possibly sleep is not improving either. To continue to make progress and ingrain a healthy transition away from parental input, we need to start phasing the parent out of the room as the child starts to feel safer and secure in the overall context of their sleep. We can do this by following the stages below.

STAGE 1: NIGHTS 1, 2, 3 AND 4

Stay beside the cot – down on the floor, ideally, at your child's level, to try to prevent standing or sitting. If they are still in the mid-level position of the cot and not mobile, then you may sit on a stool or chair.

Use the stay-and-support settling techniques outlined earlier in this chapter – physically, verbally and emotionally attending to your child. But as the first few nights pass, I would encourage you to do less – less touching, less talking, less intervention – so that we are further weakening the input need and avoiding creating new or additional sleep associations.

Lucy Says

When you begin, you may never envisage that doing less is a possibility, but this is a symbiotic relationship: the less you do, the less they will need. Your child will start to feel confident without so much support from you. Don't forget they are designed to do this – you just need to create the space!

If you continue to over-help as the first few nights elapse, then your child may cry more as you move away from the cot in the following nights, so do consciously pull back once the first two or so nights are under your belt.

Q Who should start the process, Mum or Dad?

For breastfed babies, I suggest the non-feeding parent does bedtime on nights one and two. Then Mum can do bedtime on nights three and four – wearing a newly laundered top. Overnight, it will be easier on breastfed babies if the non-feeding parent largely manages the night and Mum just appears for the feed. If your baby is not breastfed, then just decide on one parent do bedtime nights one and two and the other nights three and four. Share the load – ideally night on, night off, whatever works best for you.

Overnight plan: When your child wakes, respond immediately when you hear them, return them to the bedtime position and repeat this exercise in line with the decisions you have made about night-time feeds and other changes you are making. This becomes your new default approach to weaken the cycle of waking. See Chapter 12 to really help you work through this.

STAGE 2: NIGHTS 5, 6 AND 7

Now move to the middle of the room – sit on the chair you have been using or lie down somewhere between the cot and the door, where they can still see and hear you. Even if the room is not that big, just move slightly further away from where you started.

- Do your bedtime routine as normal, then position yourself further away from the cot.
- You can still reassure your child using the initial strategies, but more remotely. Continue to prompt verbally and always go over to physically reassure. Spend no more than 30 seconds to one minute beside the cot, then return to your new position so that ultimately they fall asleep, but now with you a little bit further away.
- If you are spending more time beside the cot than in your new position, then you are possibly doing too much and your child will become hysterical as you move further out of the room. Be there for them, relying more on your verbal reassurance than touch. Pat the mattress rather than your child. In this case, less is more.
- If your child is more upset than you would like, then you can return to being beside the cot, but you need to practise doing less of everything so moving becomes a possibility in another night or two.

Q I have started and it's going reasonably well, but I don't think my child's ready for me to move away.

Trust your judgement, remain beside the cot for nights five, six and seven and then move to stage 2. Try not to wait longer than this, though, as it may undermine the night work.

Q How will I know when they're ready for me to move away?

That's very individual. Rather than looking for signs of readiness, after the first week, I would encourage you to start moving away as above and responding as outlined below, even if they find it a bit more challenging on the first few nights of the changed position. Always remember the expected outcome is to be able to put your child into their cot and not stay with them. This work is creating the opportunity for this outcome and reducing the risk of an incomplete sleep ability that may undermine your sleep goals.

Overnight plan: You may find that at bedtime the transition is acceptable but overnight you still need to be beside the cot or bed in stage 1, as your child requires a higher level of input here. In the short term do so, but keep in mind that, ideally, overnight you will echo the same position, and definitely try to catch up by nights eight to ten onwards.

When your child wakes, give them a couple of minutes before you respond – they may surprise you and go back to sleep without you. If not, **return to your stage 1 position** and repeat this exercise. Night feeds will be now removed, if applicable, and you will repeat this approach as necessary.

STAGE 3: NIGHTS 8, 9 AND 10

Move near to the door, still lying or sitting down, still inside the room but further away again, where your child can see and hear you. If this is not possible, then my preference would be that for these days of the process your child *can still* see you, so consider moving to a position further away again, but not near the door – this will depend on the layout of the room. Do *not* move the cot once the process has started – only ever move *your* position.

- Operate as you have been, really reducing the amount of intervention.
- If you have been continually singing, now is the time to start scaling it back.
- If you have been back and forth to the cot like a yo-yo, then start to pace yourself: wait two to three minutes or more before you go back over to the cot-side and then return to the door-frame position until your child has gone to sleep.

Overnight plan: Repeat the strategies above as required. This time, though, wait longer before you return to the room – three, five or seven minutes – as your child's skill of returning to sleep will be emerging. When you go to your child overnight, keep touch and conversation to a minimum, and if it is a dummy re-plug, guide hand to mouth, or put it into their hand and leave.

Lucy Says

Avoid re-plugging the dummy and tucking the blanket or stroking the forehead, as this may become an enabler and continue to promote night-time activity.

STAGE 4: NIGHTS 11, 12 AND 13

Move out into the hallway where your child can still see and hear you, provided light and noise are not an issue. If light is a problem, then you will need to either isolate the hallway lighting or pull over the door to stop the light entering the room and overstimulating your child. The door being closed will never be important to this process, as we never want to use fear as a motivator.

- Prevent light from the hallway spilling into the bedroom; close all the other bedroom doors and black out the hall window if applicable.

- Do your bedtime routine and then move outside of the bedroom. Stand or sit at the door where your child can see and hear you.
- If you need to re-enter the room, do so on your schedule, not their demands: try four to five minutes and then increase the time gradually. Hum or shush from the door.
- Remain in position until they have gone to sleep.

Overnight plan: Ideally, overnight wakening will be really diminishing now. If it's still happening, return to the room and resume your position, but make sure that you are waiting five to seven minutes or so before responding. Many parents will now know the difference between the cry that will go back to sleep and the one that still requires you. What you may experience at this stage is a better night, but with an early start.

STAGE 5: NIGHTS 14, 15 AND 16

Move into the hallway, where your child can still hear you but not see you, and re-enter the room as necessary on a paced basis.

- Move out of view now. Either take a side step or hover in the hallway or corridor outside your child's room.
- Go into your bedroom, put away some laundry etc., letting your child hear you.
- Return to the door frame or room if you need to, briefly reassure them and leave again.
- If your child understands, tell them you will come back to check on them and make sure that you do.

Overnight plan: If your child does wake overnight, return to their room, briefly reassure them and leave again, as at bedtime.

STAGE 6: NIGHT 17 ONWARDS

Come and go as needed, over time working your way downstairs or to the living space, filling up your dishwasher (or having a glass of wine or a chocolate bar – my own preference!), observing and listening to your child on the monitor if you are using one.

Overnight plan: If your child does wake overnight – and I am hoping that this is diminishing – then give them some time to resettle themselves and, as needed, return to the room, briefly resettle them and leave. Repeat as required, always giving them plenty of space to return to sleep. Kids make lots of noise when they sleep overnight, so you may still hear them, but they don't need you. Now start to look at what you can do to help preserve your sleep – turning down the monitor, closing your bedroom door. If they need you, you will know!

Q How will I know it is working?

Typical outcomes, although all children will be different, may be that over the first few nights bedtime starts to get easier and better, with reduced or no crying. If this is not happening, review timings between bedtime and the final nap, ensure the last feed is finished at least 45 minutes before bedtime and that your child is not getting relaxed on this feed. Extend your bedtime routine and go earlier.

Overnight, I would still expect your child to wake and require resettling, but if everything is going well, as early as night 7 or more likely nights 10–14, you will experience less waking, quicker returns to sleep and a more rested child. Continue to review the changes and the timings. Observe their eating structure and milk intake. Make sure that your child is not too cold in the core part of the night. Make sure you are moving through the stages outlined.

It may take your child a while to return to sleep overnight with the new approach – it doesn't matter how long, it only matters that they return to sleep using this strategy, thus allowing it to become easier.

If you are still using a dummy then the amount of times you need to re-plug should shrink over the course of 14 nights, until you are perhaps experiencing zero to three re-plugs overnight, which for a dummy user is normal, with the expectation of improving that in the next month or so.

If you find that your child is not tolerant of you moving away, it may indicate that you have still been doing too much, so return to stage 1 and see if you can be beside your child but doing very little, so that when you try to move again it is more acceptable.

You may find your child is tolerant to you going as far as the door, but they are not open to you leaving. This is a tough one to call. For me, it should never be sleep at all costs, and you need to decide what you can commit to in this moment. If being present is what your child needs, then operate in this way for a while and postpone leaving to a later date. Obviously, if your sleep overnight is improving, then staying is not the worst presentation and nothing is forever. The only time it becomes relevant is if the night sleep is not improving. This may mean that your being there at bedtime is contributing to the night activity. Or staying may be impractical, as you may have other children that cannot be left unsupervised or it is just not an option for you or your family to stay while this child goes to sleep. In that case, you will just need to power through the upset – ensuring that all the other guides are being implemented as outlined and that you are open to this and any potential upset at this stage of the process.

Changing the approach

Some children find the parent gradually leaving too much to cope with – I describe them as all-or-nothing kind of kids – and this alone overstimulates them and makes it harder for them to settle. If this is the case, then you may need to reconsider if stay-and-support is the right approach for your child.

My main objective is to provide parents with an alternative to controlled crying and cry-intensive methods. One of the disadvantages of this approach, though, is that your child may be overstimulated by your presence. It's a chance I am prepared to take so the sleep issues can be managed as gently and sensitively as possible, but it can undermine some children's progress. If this is the case for you, then you can always revert to an interval-visit approach, as outlined on the next page – but only do this when you have completed at least seven days of my primary approach, and you are making an informed choice that this will be best for your child.

INTERVAL VISITS

With this change in approach, we will give your child a few minutes unassisted, without a parent present, so they may find their sleep ability and are not frustrated by you being there but not doing what you used to.

I suggest that you return to your child at set intervals. Begin with 5 minutes to start, then 10 minutes and then every 15 minutes until your child falls asleep.

If 5 minutes feels too long to wait, start with a smaller waiting period. But the more frequent check-ins may cause more crying. Decide what is best and stick with that – be consistent with the time frame you pick: don't wait ten minutes and then go back to five or three minutes.

To do this:

- Follow your bedtime routine as outlined earlier, with the appropriate timing. Put your child into the cot awake then leave the room.
- Wait for 5 minutes (or your decided first check-in interval).
- When it is time for the first check-in, go halfway into your child's room – so they can see you and hear you but not close enough to touch. Say something like, 'Sleep time now, I'll check on you in a while', 'Shush' or your own mantra. Your voice should be positive and loving.
- If necessary, at the start you can go over to them and touch them briefly, but very quickly stop physical intervention and rely more on a verbal and visual visit.
- Leave the room and begin the waiting interval again.
- The second interval to wait is 10 minutes (or whatever you have decided it should be). Then check in again using your voice and presence to support your child.
- The third interval, 15 minutes, is the longest you'll have to wait – you'll continue to check in at this interval.
- Repeat the process as long as needed, waiting 15 minutes, until your child falls asleep.

Key points:

- Wait the exact interval you've set for your check-ins.
- Limit the touch to your child, but be aware this might frustrate them further and they may become more upset.
- Stay just 30 seconds to 1 minute maximum before you leave again.
- If your child cries harder when you check in, you may want to extend the time between your check-ins by an additional few minutes.
- Watch for sleep cues: if your child is fussing or complaining – but not crying or crying intermittently (pauses for more than 30 seconds) – try to wait even if it is time for a check-in. This is a sign your child is learning their sleep ability and your revisit will likely interrupt the process. If they begin crying again, restart your visits using the last interval time you used. For example, if you were to check in after 10 minutes but didn't as your child was only fussing at the check-in time, but now your child is crying again, restart the timer and check in after 10 minutes.
- When your child awakens during the night, begin the process again, starting with the first interval.
- If your child is sitting or standing when you enter the room, put them down once after the second interval visit.

Lucy Says

This approach is certainly potentially a more cry-intense approach on paper and not a first choice for me as practitioner, but it suits some children better. It seems more aggressive, but this is often not the case when you swap from the initial gradual retreat as outlined. Obviously, don't do anything you are not happy with, but also serve your child well in this regard.

Chapter 4
Getting Started

When I decided to write a book based on the questions that parents ask, it became clear that there is no end to the queries that arise and it is an almost unending task. However, certain questions routinely come up, and here are my answers to those questions you may have before getting started.

Q *My baby was born prematurely – would you work from their actual or corrected age?*

Generally, I adjust to reflect the corrected age, especially when I am starting to make changes to a child's sleeping pattern. I would not normally want parents to begin a sleep-learning exercise until their child is six months corrected, and what I usually find is that, once we are making progress, most children born early fall in between their actual and their corrected age.

As they get older this matters less, as the range for the ages tends to encompass both the adjusted and actual age in the same one – it is more relevant within the first nine months, where I tend to categorise in the following ways: 0–2 months; 2–4 months; 4–6 months; 6–8 months; and then 8–12 months; 12–15 months; and 15 months–3 years. You can see that once they are beyond 8 months, they will mostly fall into the same range either way.

Q When should I begin the sleep plan?

When you start working on the initial sleep plan, starting on a Friday so that you have the weekend and, the following week, drafting in supports like a grandparent, au pair, babysitter or friend to collect other children from school for you, if applicable, is a good idea. You might look at adjusting work schedules for a few days that week for either parent, if feasible, so you have support, especially at the start.

In time, you can work on delaying nap one to after the school run or for your child to have nap one on the go – but before you can establish anything you need to go backwards to go forwards. That first 7–10 days of embedding the detail is crucial. When you have a 'working model', you can be much more flexible, and almost everything is possible, but only once your child is overall better rested.

Room-sharing

Q Where is the best place for my baby to sleep?

Where your baby sleeps is ultimately up to you. For all children, the health agenda supports room-sharing with the parent for at least the first six months, especially as you implement the sleeping-shaping foundation. After that, personal preferences apply. If you plan to move your child into their own room *and* work begin the sleep-learning exercise, then do this at the very start. A parent can share the child's room for the first three to four nights or until the parent feels emotionally ready for the child to sleep on their own.

When they're in their own room, I recommend using a monitor, but consider turning it down at night so their every movement does not wake you.

Wherever your child sleeps, spend non-sleep time in the bedroom with them and play games in the cot to help them learn that it is a safe space.

If you continue to room-share due to personal preference or space needs, then move the cot(s) as far away from the bed as possible and understand that the risks of waking each other are higher – but also the sleep disruption in attending to them is potentially less.

Wherever you decide for them to sleep, don't make any further changes after you have started making my sleep-plan adjustments for at least a month or more – don't even move the cot! Anything can potentially derail you as you start.

Q *We are keen for our children to share the same room – what are your thoughts?*

FOR MULTIPLES

Multiples room-sharing is generally a good idea, although initially it may appear that they wake each other. My experience is that they *do* sleep better together ultimately, but they need to learn to sleep *within* the noise of each other. They seem to have that skill much better than siblings!

When you are helping multiples to sleep better, I generally follow my feeding and sleeping balances and sleep plan with them at the same time and then, when necessary, I wake them within 15 minutes of each other in the morning and at naptime, so we can have the same day routine and bedtime for both. I find twins will synchronise then thereafter.

Ideally, twins in the same room means that you can have one bedtime and naptime routine carried out by one parent. I like having the cots parallel to each other, where they can see and hear each other. If you are starting the sleep-learning approach, then it is better if both parents or at least two adults take a child each at the start, until you move to stage 2 – then one parent can do everything. I like the outcome for families with multiples to be: one parent, one bedroom (if desirable), one bedtime routine, one set of twins or triplets or even quads into their respective cots or beds and then to sleep (in time, anyway).

Lucy Says

You need to commit to not taking them out of the room overnight to avoid waking each other. You will need to work through this so that they can become adjustable to each other's sounds – and sometimes annoyed by it: one boy twin that I worked with told his sister to be quiet with a big shush! They will mostly synchronise their sleeping patterns over the following few weeks with a similar napping and waking pattern.

Although, of course, I acknowledge that even though they were born at the same time they have different personalities, I do, however, put them on the same timing and sleep plan, as otherwise it would be unsustainable in the long-term for the parents. You can then ensure that you are meeting their individual needs within this framework.

FOR SIBLINGS

If you have children of different ages sharing a room and one or both or all of them have sleep challenges, then the issues are best dealt with individually.

Attempting to address often deeply ingrained sleep challenges with children of different ages, needs and abilities is far too ambitious. Even as a seasoned practitioner, I will not address two children of different ages at the same time. I suggest that you select the 'priority sleeper' – the one that perhaps is causing the most stress or contributes most to the low level of sleep that you get – and begin from there.

Very often, the changes that you make with child one somehow actually help with child two, and no action is required. But if it is, you begin again with a new sleep plan for the next child.

Ideally, although not always convenient, move them into separate rooms, even if that means one child returns to the parents' bedroom (not bed) 'on holidays' until the first sleep issues are diminished. Room-sharing is much more productive when all parties are sleep able.

Case Study

John and Aaron are two boys aged three and a half and eight months respectively. Aaron's bedtime is delayed to allow John – who does sleep well – to go to sleep and then Aaron goes up at 9 p.m. when it is safe. Unfortunately, Aaron wakes frequently at night and Mum panics, as she doesn't want to wake John, bringing Aaron out of the shared room and into the family bed. Aaron continues to wake, despite being in the bed, and now everyone is at their wits' end.

The boys must share a room due to space; however, unless the parents commit to not removing either child from the bedroom for fear of waking the other, we need to make a temporary adjustment. I recommend that, as this family begins making changes, they move John into his parents' bedroom on a camp bed or mattress, explaining that he will be having a 'holiday' in Mum and Dad's room until Aaron is sleeping better.

Now they can address Aaron's sleep issues in the room the boys will ultimately sleep in, but without delaying bedtime or worrying about waking John or ingraining a bed-share dynamic for Aaron that the parents do not want to commit to.

I would suggest they take their time addressing all the issues. Once Aaron is sleeping better and all elements feel robust – within three weeks or so – then the boys should be reunited. Depending on timings, they could have one bedtime routine for both children at the same time or, if they have different bedtimes, stagger them.

Q We have three children, and I'm not sure how to manage bedtime

Many parents' bedtime routine is challenging with more than one child. As with room-sharing and managing school runs, for example, two adults in the home is ideal at the start – one to work with the priority sleeper and one to either mind or put to bed the other child or children. Try to do this for as long as you can and then when it is necessary for one parent to manage both at the same time, you could consider one bedtime routine in the shared bedroom of both children or the bedroom of the child who was not routinely sleeping well.

At that stage, I would hope that a sleep ability has been established, and you can deposit both children to their respective cots or beds and leave the room so that trying to be in two places at one time is not necessary.

As with most parenting tasks, this is a management issue. Personally, I used to take two or three children up at the same time. I would encourage the older two to read or look at books in their own room while I tended to the youngest – then once they were in their cot, sleep ready and able, I worked my way to the others, so they each got a little bit of important one-to-one time with me before sleep.

This takes some time to master, but having a sleep-able unit makes everything more achievable.

Lucy Says

Successful room-sharing emerges when healthy boundaries are encouraged, such as no talking when lights are out, no messing, no waking another from sleep, and from trying to create that boundary very early on so you don't see a degradation of either child's sleep as time goes by.

Q We only have one bedroom – can the plan still work?

If you cannot move the children around as suggested for John and Aaron, then you will have to apply all the strategies and the overnight learning approach as needed, committing to not bringing the priority sleeper, or ideally either, out of the room unless it is morning time proper. This may mean more than one child awake temporarily, so then you'd take a child each – so you'll need the other parent or another adult drafted in to help on the first few, potentially challenging nights. Once things start to improve – and they will – the need for support from others diminishes and the changes become more movable, workable parts of the fabric of your well-rested lives.

Lucy Says

All of the above can feel initially overwhelming, but as with everything I suggest, take it in small chunks of time and slowly grow your sleep with my guidance.

Q *I have school runs – how can I fit in naps and collecting the other children?*

This is a tough one, as school runs typically seem to happen when our younger children need to nap – meaning that a high percentage of the issues you experience are because the day sleep cannot be prioritised. That does not mean that you can't work through this. Personally, I have successfully managed the 12.30/1.30 p.m. and 2.30 p.m. collections and had a happy napper and overall rested little person too. I don't want you to think that it was easy – it wasn't – but it *was* achievable and it does end!

First, the reality is that it's almost impossible to address reported sleep issues unless you initially apply my sleep timings outlined for your child's age. This does make up a large percentage of the reported issues and so demands application, at least at the start.

That said, I do find that once we begin to apply the initial timing suggestions, together with the other elements of your sleep plan, your child starts to sleep better and you achieve a 'working model'. Then you can typically adjust naps to happen after the morning and afternoon school runs.

The tricky territory is when you have one or two naps and a collection at 1.30 p.m. *and* 2.30 p.m., for example, which means there's not really anywhere to adjust the single or second nap to – as a single nap would ideally have a 1 p.m. start time and a second nap about 1.30 p.m. This really is hard and you may need to get creative, allowing this nap to be cot- or car-based, considering after-school care, activities or homework club, or asking someone to babysit for the naptime/school-run time or car-pooling with another parent in the same boat so that not every day is affected. The more rested your child becomes, the more adjustable they can also be, but not every child is willing to acclimatise. In time you will learn what suits your child best, but at least once they're well rested there is more to work with, rather than you all being sleep-deprived and starting on the back foot.

Lucy Says

When you only have the 1.30 or 2.30 p.m. school run then you can orchestrate the single nap to happen before or after, whichever is the best fit.

Daycare

Q What can I do about daycare and my childminder?

A lot of our children will be in daycare when we return to work. I always suggest that, when possible, you work on your reported sleep issues about six weeks or so before your return-to-work date so you don't run into any issues. This can be hard if you return to work when your child is six months or younger, as you may only have been able to apply my early sleep-shaping suggestions until then. However, even that is helpful to achieving later sleep goals.

For a smooth(ish) transition to crèche, try to ensure that your child is well rested and capable of sleeping, ideally with a complete sleep ability (when age relevant), before they begin their induction. Make sure you are using my age-appropriate time structure by day and that your crèche is willing, at the start, at least, to work on this with you rather than immediately adhering to their particular daytime structure.

My age-appropriate feeding and sleeping balances (see p. 95) will help you endeavour to ensure that your child is a relatively good sleeper at home before expecting them to transfer this skill to another environment. It really is important to do your best to address any sleep issues before you return to work. That way, you will be handing over a robust and well-rested child and reduce the risks of challenges further down the line.

Lucy Says

Some children will never sleep as well in a crèche as they would at home and the reverse is also true. It can take three to four weeks for your child to fully establish their sleep in the crèche, and if they have a sleep ability for naps, then this can be more easily transferred to daycare – rather than having to learn two skills they only have to master one.

Unfortunately, when most children begin their crèche induction, they may well pick up a cough or a cold as well, and this can make the mastering of crèche sleep a bit more challenging. I would hope that, as your child settles in and acclimatises to the new environment, their carers will give them some extra attention and provide the space and opportunity for them to get good at sleeping in the crèche.

Consider that not only does your child need to familiarise themselves with sleeping in a communal, often noisy and not dark enough new sleep space – they are also getting used to not being with you all day every day too! Ensure that you are spending lots of emotionally connected time with your child, and providing lots of opportunity for physical and eye contact when you are together. The quality of the time you are together should be deep and meaningful.

Lucy Says

Send a security item with your child, and a sleeping bag if you usually use one and if it is allowed, and tell the carers a few quick phrases that you say at home that they can repeat to your baby when they attempt a nap. A good sleep environment away from home would ideally be dark and without too many disruptions. If music or white noise is playing it should do so for the duration of the sleep.

You already know that settling-in issues and possibly some sickness are likely, but that will all settle down within a month in most cases. Your baby is adaptable, but you know your child best – and if they seem to take longer to adjust than others, then make sure you factor that in too.

Naps are usually short in crèche, but will increase in time – provided, of course, the sleep ability already exists.

Q My child is already in a crèche five days a week – I desperately want to improve their sleep, though, both at home and in daycare

Working on your sleep challenges and creating a sleep ability when your child is already in daycare of any description is completely doable. You will require positive input from your daycare provider to follow the plan and timings to the best of their ability as the sleep is being grown at home. It is in their best interests to help with this, as a well-rested, easy-to-put-down child is also easier to mind, teach and feed.

Older children in a crèche are very often on a single nap too early in the day – it starts possibly at about 11.45–12 and thus, even if it is an adequate duration and you are observing a suitable bedtime, the gap of wakefulness exceeds the biological sleep need as outlined in my nap-gap dynamic. This results in a host of issues for working parents.

I would love for crèche organisations to take note that the ideal biological time for a single nap is more like 1 p.m. This way the nap can also finish later, bedtime can be appropriate and the risks of waking and early rising are diminished. I salute daycares open to adjusting daytime sleep, as it has positive implications across the board, supporting positive sleep practices and child development.

Also, be mindful that if your childminder is caring for other children and also needs to do school runs, then this can negatively impact your child's sleeping pattern. Bear in mind that – in an effort to ensure that your child's sleep is future-proofed, once remedied – from 8 months to 15–18 months, two naps are typically needed. The times of these naps, when sleep ability is established, is between 9 and 9.30 a.m. and about 1.30 p.m. When your child is ready for one nap, the ideal timing is from 1 p.m.

Lucy Says

That is not to say other start and finish times don't work, but these times definitely do work. Literally thousands of families that I help report that observing the suggested biologically times are a game changer for sleep.

Wherever your child is by day – whether in crèche, with a child minder or with Granny – whoever is managing day sleep should be:

- Timing it as outlined
- Creating a sleep-inducing environment
- Prioritising your child's individual needs for sleep in the main

Q *My child is always getting sick. We make progress but then we find ourselves back at square one*

Sickness and teething have an ongoing impact on your child's ability to sleep well. Many children will experience bouts of routine illnesses such as ear, throat and chest infections, colds and viruses with minimum sleep disturbance. Others will have parents up at night as they work their way through feeling under the weather, and very often for a few weeks after the illness has passed. Children who are only just learning to sleep better will definitely be more vulnerable during this time.

Lucy Says

Only start to address your child's sleep ability when they are 100 per cent well. Don't delay starting due to teething (or any other developmental leap), as your child will teethe on and off for over two years. Don't, though, start when they are visibly teething – see symptoms below – or slightly under the weather.

If your child gets sick when you are mid sleep plan, then you can expect to not make progress at the anticipated rate and it will be potentially more difficult to stay on track, both emotionally and physically.

In terms of sickness, in my experience it can often take 7–10 days *after* the antibiotic/medication is finished before you start to see improved sleep re-emerging, and sometimes even longer.

To expect better sleep or to get back on track, then, your child will need to be completely well and symptom-free, off any medication, with restored appetite and improved mood and behaviour. It can often be helpful to return to the doctor for a review and confirmation that they are better. That being the case, it will still potentially take more time to get back to where you were.

Lucy Says

If you have been experiencing improvement and there's a sudden deterioration then this is often the first indicator of a sickness or teething period.

Some subtle changes that may indicate your child is teething or starting to come down with something are:

- Temperature
- Off food
- Change in mood or behaviour
- Uncharacteristic crying or clingy behaviour
- Messy nappies
- Constipation
- Flushed cheeks
- Sore bottom
- Excessive drooling

- Untypical frequent night waking, sleep resistance, short naps, early awakening (when you had made progress)

You will probably see symptoms of teething during the day, not just at night. However, it will definitely be more pronounced at night, when there are no distractions, and when the child is lying down.

Lucy Says

During a period of sickness or teething, I would encourage parents to have a response plan so that you don't operate a crisis-management approach to the sleep challenges that may undermine your previous hard work and linger long after the sickness itself.

Unfortunately, reintroducing previous sleep associations can quickly re-establish them – in as little as one to three days – so it is important to manage a sick or teething phase appropriately, understanding that during this time no one is going to get much sleep anyway.

Even a talented sleeper may be knocked off course by sickness or teething, so if you are mid-cycle of a sleep-learning exercise it will be even more challenging and disheartening. Try not to worry. Focus on your goals and how far you have already come and operate as follows:

- Use medication and pain reliever as directed by your GP.
- Be responsive at all times and don't allow your baby to cry when unwell. A pain cry is often high-pitched and constant and may not come under control immediately on pick-up. Protest crying, although high-pitched with some children, is generally not constant and can be stopped immediately on pick-up.
- If you are not typically bed-sharing or plan to commit to this, or have recently reversed this cycle, then it may not be the best idea to bring your child back into your bed when sick or teething. Very quickly they may start to prefer your sleep environment to theirs and then wake at night to be brought back in again long after sickness or teething has passed. I suggest camping out in *their* bedroom so you can supervise and monitor your child if they are significantly under the weather.

- If you have weaned night-time feeds, then try not to go back there. Offer a sippy cup of water to keep them hydrated, but stop this as soon as they're feeling better as this, too, can quickly become anticipated every night.
- If in doubt about intake and you have night-weaned, then you could always provide a dream feed (see page 77) around 10–11.30 p.m. You initiate this and wake your child so you don't re-engage the expectation to feed at night, but you do ensure they get what they need during this time frame.
- If they are very unsettled overnight, it can sometimes help to get up for a while – go downstairs but don't turn on the lights or TV – just take a break, give meds as appropriate and then return to bed with a routine to help them go back to sleep.
- Make sure that during a sick or teething period you observe a relatively early bedtime: 6–7 p.m. is often best.
- You can let them nap more but always curtail nap one to an hour and a half and finish the day for naps as outlined for your age group.
- Try to keep the 'new way' of going to sleep in place, even if you need to support them more or go back to stage 1. Do this and when they are better quickly get back to where you were and resume the learning cycle.
- Provide extra reassurance at bedtime and overnight as appropriate – you may find that overnight is very challenging so just do your best to support them. It will start to improve again once they feel better.
- Make sure they are well rested during the day – if they are cot-resistant then perhaps use the back-up plan of the car, buggy, couch and so on until they are back to themselves.

As soon as your child starts to recover – good indicators would be completion of their antibiotic/medication, improved mood and behaviour, back on their food – then I would try to work your way back to where you were. Routinely, post-sickness or teething, many parents find their sleep improvements return – their child goes to sleep easily and starts to stay asleep again. Others may find their child is more clingy and needy. Once you are confident they are 100 per cent well, you may need to implement stage 1 onwards to restore good sleep.

Lucy Says

I find it can often take a child three to four weeks post-sickness to get back to good sleep, so give them a chance without being aggressive, and view this challenging time as part of our journey as parents.

[Q] *I have a dummy – do I need to get rid of it?*

If your child is aged between six and nine months and still has a dummy then, with GP consent, you could drop it at bedtime as you start making changes and replace it with the stay-and-support approach.

If your child is more upset than you would like when you do this, then return the dummy and understand that your child is not a willing participant in the withdrawal and you cannot do it without the dummy at this time.

If your child is older than nine months, or if you plan to keep the dummy, then you can still get great sleep. Yes, you may need to help them find the dummy here and there, but you can teach them to use it – always put it into their hand and guide the hand to their mouth. Over time, help their hand look for it by swiping it about the cot.

If they throw out the dummy to get you to return or to get your attention, then make sure to have spares in your pocket – don't react, wait three to five minutes, give a new dummy and retrieve the other one at a later stage.

Lucy Says

I'm not a fan of more than one dummy at a time, so just get good with one before you bring substitutes on the pitch.

Chapter 5

Birth to Four Months

Becoming a new parent is both exhilarating and overwhelming in equal measure. We cannot underestimate the adjustment required when we bring a human into our world. Whether it is the first time or the fifth time, each parenting journey comes with joy but also with challenges. Each tiny individual will respond to the world in a different way and you may find that what worked for your first baby does not with your second. Or you may find that your parenting experience is just not what you expected or anticipated. You may find yourself lacking in confidence, second-guessing yourself and feeling like you are doing everything wrong. This is very normal, but nonetheless challenging. Some of you will find yourself in circumstances that are (un)planned – parenting alone or with the other parent living away for work some or all of the week. So many changes are happening to your body and to your life as you knew it. Time for yourself is a distant memory and connected time as a couple feels very remote. Of course, the good nearly always outweighs the bad, but it is hard, and when you struggle with sleep you are not operating at your optimal level, while also trying to deal with the many new feelings and emotions that can arise when you become a parent. Please seek support and guidance when appropriate and be open to asking for help in whatever form is available – your GP, health visitor, partner, friends, family and so on.

Lots of new babies don't exactly 'sleep like a baby' and you may find that you struggle to get them to sleep and to stay asleep for any length of time. This is considered typical infant behaviour and not a problem that requires intervention. Certainly there are adjustments you can try and discoveries you may need to make – for example, are there underlying medical barriers contributing to the reported problems: digestive issues, reflux, food sensitivities, tongue tie, feeding issues? There are so many factors that can affect your journey that I alone cannot always address them. To that end, I have interviewed a number of experts in Chapter 15, who shed some light on their disciplines and what you can do to help support yourself and your baby on this tricky journey. Their valuable input, together with my own recommendations, will hopefully help you to not only survive but thrive, and feel heard, supported and empowered as a parent too.

Q My baby will only sleep in my arms

This is probably the most common report I receive from parents of newborns. Parents explain that their new baby will only settle when they are being held. When they try to place them down in their sleeper, they either wake immediately or within a short period of time. If held, however, they may stay asleep, but this means that busy parents can get nothing done and, of course, overnight sleep is elusive and safe sleep may be compromised too.

First, babies are born with a high need to be held. They have been held *in utero* for nine months, and in the outside world, their need to be close to the parent, in arms, and to be rocked and shushed, similar to in the womb, still exists. We often refer to this period as the fourth trimester – your baby was physically ready to be born but developmentally is not ready to be separate from you. They rely solely on you for their every need and are extremely vulnerable. I recommend that you lean into this need – that you hold, rock and cuddle with your baby – and suggest that your task in these early days and months is to teach your baby to feel loved, safe and secure and that there will be a response from you every time. It is a loving trust-building exercise.

They need you for food, love, comfort, warmth, connection and so on – and if you can meet these needs, then their trust and belief in you will rise, their confidence on the outside world will grow and their ability to be more separate from you will also expand, as they get older, knowing they can rely on you. This sets the scene for your child's ongoing development and their bonded relationship with you, and while you are doing this, I believe you can work behind the scenes, enabling a foundation for positive sleep practices too.

I do not believe in the concept of bad habits, spoiling babies or making a rod for your own back. I do not believe that you can be manipulated or played by them. I believe that this relationship must be loving, emotionally connected and fulfilling, that unmet needs create untold issues and that, even if you could spoil a baby, then this is what must happen as you help them learn to live in the world.

Accepting this, however tiring and challenging, is setting the tone for your parent–child relationship for all time. Meet their needs with speed and with love. Understand their needs and honour your own too, such as asking for help and support, sharing the load between both parents, if applicable, and creating space to maintain your own unique being, while you cultivate the relationship and grow with your child.

Needing to be held is not a problem; it does not require intervention or to be fixed. It is just a typical infant tendency. Accept this and in the background start to make some adjustments that can help your child's sleep ability emerge over time.

Sleep shaping

Observe a flexible feeding and sleeping framework to your day. From perhaps six weeks onwards, follow the feeding and sleeping balances set out in Chapter 8. The most important elements here would be a regular wake time no later than 7.30 a.m. and to start the day with a feed – separate to sleep – exposing baby to bright and/or natural light when possible.

Q *My baby won't take a feed first thing in the morning as they have fed not too long ago in the night-time period*

It is important to be able to anchor the day with a regular wake time to hormonally regulate the biological time clock and to synchronise your baby's feeds for the day. That way your feeding rhythm and sleeping rhythm will be in sync with each other and this can make feeding and sleeping easier for you as the day unfolds. If, due to a feed earlier in the night, you cannot establish the morning feed, perhaps consider a smaller night-time feed at 3–5 a.m., or just one breast, to try to observe this practice.

Q *Is it too soon for a routine?*

Knowing, as we do, that sleep challenges can be born of biological timekeeping issues, I believe that as soon as you feel able, possibly from six weeks onwards – once your feeding practice is established and you have had your six-week check-up – you can start to shape your day with some subtle adjustments. Observe the framework detailed below and do your best to meet your baby's needs for sleep, feeding and connection.

Ideally, your baby will feed by day every 1–3 hours, depending on your chosen feeding practice, but they will also need to sleep every 1–2 hours and you are, without putting yourself or the baby under undue pressure, trying to create a balance between the two. Remember, the timings are just a guide, not a rigid prescription – it is early days and so expectations of what baby can achieve should be low.

Lucy Says

In the first few weeks your feeding practice will take precedence over sleep – if breastfeeding, you will just be focused on your supply, your position and ensuring that baby is getting enough milk and, regardless of breast or bottle, that connection and comfort are prioritised.

As your baby gets a little older, allowing sleep and feeding to have almost equal importance is key. Childhood development is not one-dimensional – ensuring that your child is well rested at the right time for the body and well fed and always feels loved can lead to better outcomes for all involved.

Q *I have heard about sleep cues, but I really am not sure what to look out for*

Learning to read your baby's language for sleep is key. Being responsive to your baby's sleep cues or signals in the early months has proven to have positive outcomes, and are considered to be the first steps towards positive sleep practices. Early sleep cues are brief, but when acted on, can mean that your baby may go to sleep with ease and stay asleep for longer.

Typical early sleep cues may be represented by eye rubs, yawns, moments of quiet where baby zones out momentarily or snuggles away from you. These early signals mean that the body is getting ready for sleep, hormonally and chemically, and given the opportunity may fall asleep quickly and achieve a deeper, more rested sleep.

Late sleep cues are more obvious and ideally avoided – they may be represented by intense eye rubbing, big yawns, a sense of agitation – clenching the fists, stretching the limbs, arching the back, whinging, being fussy, moaning and/or starting to cry. These cues mean the body has had a chemical reaction – cortisol and adrenaline are now in the system and we are in fight-or-flight mode. This makes falling asleep much more challenging, as the body now resists it. It may also mean that staying asleep is difficult, resulting in short bursts of sleep rather than longer nap durations if able.

If you never seem to see the early sleep signals, then it can be worth keeping a diary and attempting a nap 10–20 minutes before you usually see the late cues.

Lucy Says

Typically, after waking in the morning as outlined, the wake period before nap 1 is really quite small, 45–75 minutes. Observing this small wake period and then not allowing baby to be awake for more than one and a half to two hours at any one time can create better opportunities for avoiding overtiredness and encouraging more rest for your baby.

Even if sleep is only in your arms, in the buggy, sling or the car (all used as per the manufacturers' safety guidelines), this will help ensure that your baby does not routinely repeat an overtired cycle. Overtired babies tend to be fussy and not stay on the task of feeding when offered, leading to a 'drip' feed or 'grazing' feeding dynamic.

Q My baby will only nap for 10–40 minutes at a time – I really want him to sleep for 1–2 hours!

Managing expectations is key in the early months. Your child's nap rhythms are immature until six months plus, so the ability to nap for longer durations varies hugely. Have no expectation of nap duration, and this way you will avoid unnecessary frustration. Know that applying my feeding and sleeping balances to your day is encouraging a longer nap when your child is ready to do so. If all they do is 20–30 minutes, then just get up and move on, ensuring that you feed them when needed and you attempt a nap again within an hour and a half to two hours of waking. If after only napping for a short period of time baby seems tired again soon, then allow at least an hour to an hour and a half to pass before attempting another nap, as sleep pressure needs to be adequate for another nap to actually happen. Avoid putting yourself under unnecessary pressure – many parents spend too much time in the early months stressing about sleep that is just not ready or able to emerge, but it will: just continue to work behind the scenes.

Percentage-of-wakefulness approach

Q You suggest that feeding or holding to sleep can become a contributory factor in sleep issues. How can I help to prevent my baby being entirely asleep on the last feed at bedtime?

Despite wanting to be in your arms and held by you or needing lots of motion or a rocking action to encourage sleep by day and at night, when your baby is going to sleep at bedtime there is an ideal opportunity to lessen this desire, without compromising baby's needs, and to help take a greater, closer step in the direction of enhanced sleep ability.

The percentage-of-wakefulness approach is best used from six to eight weeks until twelve weeks or so. The sooner you can start to implement it, the more open your baby may be to learning. Knowing that, in time, holding and rocking and feeding to sleep can become a core contributory reason behind some of the reported sleep issues that parents experience, at bedtime specifically, when the sleep drive is strong, we can practise having your baby a little bit more awake and a little bit less asleep when they are placed wherever you would like baby to sleep overnight.

Using this approach at bedtime creates awareness and sleep ability. Your baby is cognisant they have been put down, even in a small capacity, and this action means that when they start to cycle through sleep in an adult-orientated way (from four months onwards) then they are more likely to sleep through their natural sleep phases and only wake when hungry, need brief connection with you or have had enough sleep. This may prevent them from waking unnecessarily, as the brain learns early on to get through the phases of sleep, and all of this learning can be achieved at bedtime proper.

In the first few months, your baby's bedtime is really quite late. It is your bedtime, in essence. This is the fertile ground to help them learn to be put down out of arms – using their hormonally strong drive to sleep and their final milk feed for now. In the early months your final milk feed *will* accompany sleep. You will see later that I adjust this if we are struggling with reported issues overnight, but in the first six months milk and sleep go together at bedtime and there is no need to create the large distance I suggest later on. You may think, why not do this now? Well, we are still relying on milk to help induce sleep and keep your baby asleep as long as possible in the early months – sleep is still immature and we are just preparing for the maturation.

If you prepare in the early months, then you may never need to create distance between the last feed and sleep, as the brain has been given the learning opportunity early on and this alone may encourage the deeper, less interrupted sleep – and if it doesn't, then we adjust things from six months onwards when sleep is formed and the opportunity to developmentally evolve your child's sleep truly exists.

The percentage-of-wakefulness approach is essentially having your baby 'drowsy but awake' – I find this terminology too subjective, as what is drowsy to you may be entirely different to me and the next parent and so on. So I use 'percentage of wakefulness' because it is visual too.

At the start your baby is likely to be 100 per cent asleep on the last feed at bedtime, which will be quite late. You will now be going up to your bedroom, to a sleep-friendly environment, and preparing baby to sleep with a pre-sleep ritual.

For example, enter the room, dim the light, close the curtains, repeat a sleep phrase, sing a familiar song, get your baby changed and then start to feed. Before they fall 100 per cent asleep on either the breast or the bottle, unlatch or detach, wind, cuddle and place in the sleeper maybe 95 per cent asleep and 5 per cent aware that you put them down. Stroke and shush them as they complete going to sleep, and acknowledge that this act alone is enabling sleep ability for the months to follow. As time goes by, practise improving the percentage ratio to 90/10, 80/20, 70/30 and so on. The more awake they are at bedtime once placed in the crib, the higher the chance of sleeping deeper and longer with reduced interruptions. You are creating space and opportunity for the brain to learn to get to sleep without too much intervention from you, and this unlocks the ability that can then be transferred into the daytime sleep ability overtime.

Lucy Says

If you are using a dummy, try to remove it from the mouth before they're entirely asleep. If they continue to suck, push up their chin and stroke and rub them, so sucking to sleep does not become the only way your baby can get through night-time phases of sleep. Understand that you may always need to help your child with their dummy as explained earlier (see page 57).

Q *I have tried this approach with my baby, but unless they are 100 per cent asleep, they cry and will not settle*

This approach needs to be implemented with little or no crying, so if you try this, having observed the feeding and sleeping balances for your child's age as detailed, and if you are preparing the sleep environment, providing the pre-sleep ritual and trying to have them less asleep but they won't tolerate it and only cry, then stop tonight, hold, rock, feed to sleep – but do try again in another few days or within a week. It may be that your baby is just not developmentally able or ready for this separation, albeit small, and you need to meet them where they are at.

We don't want any crying to sleep at this early age, and we don't want to encourage sleep at your child's expense: they need to be ready and some are just not. Keep trying, however, and, more importantly, keep observing all the other elements that support better sleep, and if by four months your baby is still not open to percentage of wakefulness, commit to the rocking or feeding until six months plus, and then we can change the approach to a sleep-learning exercise when they may be more ready to embrace sleep ability.

Q *I have noticed that my baby is getting tired earlier in the evening in the last week or so*

As your baby gets older, their bedtime shifts earlier, so by around four months bedtime ranges between 6 and 8 p.m. – do your best here now to follow the nap-gap dynamic outlined (see page 174) and avoid the wake period before bedtime exceeding two hours. The aim is largely to be asleep by 7 p.m. once baby is sixteen weeks plus.

Lucy Says

When we do not bring bedtime forward early enough then we may find that the longer sleep stretches you were establishing start to disappear. This indicates the biological need to achieve sleep earlier as your baby gets older. Dismissing this can lead to unwanted sleep challenges for your family.

Overnight

Q *How do I deal with my baby overnight?*

Really, there is no plan for the nights in the early months – if your baby wakes and is due or requires a feed, then provide this as appropriate. If they wake and want to be with you, then embrace night-time parenting and meet baby where they are at. Although *we* are used to sleeping overnight, they are not, and you may find that they sleep and feed and then stay awake for a good while and return to sleep after an hour or two. This may be frustrating, but knowing it is typical is helpful.

Lucy Says

Overnight, keep your baby in the bedroom that you sleep in. Keep the lights low and avoid overstimulating them, although do not avoid engagement with them. Avoiding eye contact together with refusing emotional or physical support could make your baby feel anxious and search out more support from you – so lean into loving them back overnight, even though you would prefer to be asleep. This time will pass – soon enough they will sleep for longer and wake less often.

Remember to:

- Keep the lights low.
- Don't remove them from the room for feeds or anything else.
- Change the nappy as needed, keeping disruption to a minimum.
- Engage with but don't stimulate them so much as to give mixed messages about what happens overnight, but don't withdraw support either.
- Return them to their sleeper as appropriate.
- If you are bed-sharing, then ensure that you are making an informed decision and creating a safe sleep environment for you and your family.

Q *Although we didn't plan to, I am more and more bringing baby into bed with me*

Many families will practise bed-sharing at some point in their parenting career. I personally enjoyed bed-sharing with my breastfed babies and found it a good way to achieve the greatest amount of undisrupted sleep. That said, it is not supported by the health agenda, and so families who opt for it, either as part of a parenting style or reactively as a means to helping everyone sleep some more, may often feel unsupported.

Whatever your decision, it is important that, even in the fog of sleep deprivation, you are still making informed decisions around where your baby will sleep.

- Always place baby on a firm, clean surface under breathable bedding.
- Remove loose bedding, stuffed toys and pillows.
- Ensure there are no gaps or spaces that present a risk for getting trapped or suffocation.
- Ensure a smoke-free home.
- Avoid falling asleep in a chair or sofa.
- All parties sharing the bed have equal responsibility – never bed-share having taken alcohol or medication.

For more information, please see the co-sleeping guidelines at cosleeping.nd.edu. For general SIDS awareness for all children, see the overview of cot death at www2.hse.ie.

Daytime sleep

Q *Where do you suggest my baby sleeps during the day?*

If you are making progress at bedtime, you may now be able to attempt nap 1 or nap 2 in the sleeper with a similar approach, although it is unlikely you will have a bottle or breastfeed just before naptime according to my feeding and sleeping suggestions, which say to have feeds between sleeps rather than always just before. However, having established correct timing, take your baby to the bedroom for the nap. Use a pre-sleep ritual – dim the lights, put baby into their swaddle or sleeping sack, sing songs, cuddle and say familiar phases, place them in the sleeper and stroke and rub them to sleep. In time, reduce this activity so their ability to do this themselves is continually enhanced.

Lucy Says

In recent times, swaddling has been discouraged, following some studies that indicated unsafe swaddling practices were leading to issues with displaced hips, for example. Many babies, though, do appreciate the feeling of being wrapped. If you're comfortable doing so, you could wrap a blanket around their arms and tuck it in, but leave the lower end of the blanket loosely wrapped around their legs instead of tucking it in tightly and restricting lower-leg movement. By four months, when baby is starting to roll, a sleeping bag is preferred. Always discuss with your GP or health visitor if in any doubt.

Always create a dark environment for the nap, along with a wind-down activity. If your baby continually struggles, try going for the nap a bit sooner so they are easily able to go to sleep and not as resistant. If this is still not working, then commit to motion sleep in arms or buggy (even just rolled in the house) or the car and address this sleep segment as outlined in Chapter 14.

Q Although I am doing everything that you say, my baby just won't stay asleep for long

Once again, don't worry about duration: it is not necessarily there to be had. Concentrate on ability at the onset of sleep and the duration of sleep will catch up. If you feel your baby can be comforted back to sleep mid-nap, then that is wonderful, but I wouldn't invest too much time in it, as the ability may not be ready to emerge. Focus on all the other suggestions and have faith that beyond six months most children can be encouraged to have at least one nap of at least an hour per day.

If your child is routinely having short naps, try to have the first two naps in the cot and then just provide a series of naps on the go: car, buggy, sling, swing.

Q Is it OK for the naps to be in the pram or the car?

In the beginning, your baby is super portable, and I suggest that you let them sleep in any safe way that works for them. Best practice in time will be that nap 1 and nap 2 are ideally cot-based. This can only really be achieved if you are making progress with the bedtime sleep ability, as this skill can then be transferred into the day. Some parents will decide that they don't want naps in the cot as it is tying, but in time you may discover that for your child to ultimately sleep well, one or two of the day sleeps have to be in the cot. You will retain these naps for the first 15–18 months, and then the second nap will become the main single nap, which will be with you until three years or so. Establishing this pattern will help ensure that baby is getting not only enough sleep, but also good quality sleep, which only motionless sleep can achieve in the main.

If your child finds it very challenging to nap in the cot, use the car, buggy or swing and retry after six months of age, when the nap rhythm is more established and the cot and night-time can be worked on more intensely if necessary.

Lucy Says

If your child does not fall sleep in the cot at bedtime, with some level of awareness, it can mean that they won't be able to achieve day sleep in this way until the skill is in place at bedtime proper. In general, it is the bedtime skill set that is transferrable to the daytime.

As ever, just do your best: you are enough, and whatever challenges you experience do not mean you are doing something wrong. There is nothing more unpredictable than human behaviour – and even more unpredictable is infant human behaviour. Continue to roll with small changes and underpin your knowledge with patience, ring-fenced with a loving message.

Chapter 6

Early Routines: Birth to Four Months

Knowing, as we do, that many sleep challenges stem from timekeeping and overtiredness, then having a shape on the day can help to either avoid or reverse this dynamic for you. In the early months, this is meant to only act as a framework and not a prescriptive guide, as your baby will have their own ideas and struggles that we often just have to live with.

As your child gets older, the suggested timings are more definitive, but this is less so initially, with some children having a late bedtime for the first three to four months and others ready for the early bedtime by as young as two months. I want you to have a guide but I do not want you to become so deeply entrenched in detail that you cannot see the wood for the trees.

It will help if you keep in mind that at this early age and stage there is so much variability that often your effort doesn't deliver. But even if you are not getting a return on your investment yet, it will all pay dividends as your child becomes older and more open to the changes that you ultimately make.

Of course, early intervention is important too, as then there is less chance of having to create a sleep plan to address issues. Always work from your child's current age, and if they were premature and treated as such, then use their corrected age (see page 43).

Feeding and sleeping suggestions: up to two months

- Total amount of sleep: 14–17 hours in a 24-hour period
- Number of naps: 5–8 throughout the day
- Daytime sleep not necessarily organised, with naps from 20 minutes to 2–3 hours per sleep segment
- Don't worry about nap amounts: get the balance between the naps working well and the duration will emerge
- Feeds: every three hours for bottle, possibly more frequent for breastfed

7–7.30 a.m.	Start the day no later than 7.30 a.m., regardless of what has happened overnight
	Get out of bed and expose your baby to natural/bright light
	Provide a morning feed within the first 30 minutes of waking to anchor your day feeds, regardless of what feeds have happened overnight
7.45–9 a.m.	Prepare for your first nap within 45 minutes and no longer than 1½ hours of being awake
	Pay attention to your baby's sleep cues and act on them
	If you don't see them looking tired, prepare for the nap 10–20 minutes before the end of the suggested wake period
	This nap may be as little as 20 minutes or it may be more than an hour
	Allow your baby to wake naturally, but wake them to maintain your next feed, which will be due three hours after the first morning feed
10–10.30 a.m.	Provide a feed
	Expose to natural light
	Leisure time

11 a.m. –12 p.m.	Depending on time and duration of nap 1, prepare for the next nap within 1½–2 hours of being awake
	Be careful not to plan your sleep time according to the time your baby has fed – base it on the time your baby woke and also read their sleep cues
	This nap may be as little as 40 minutes or it may be more than an hour
	Allow your baby to wake naturally, but wake them to maintain your next feed, which will be due three hours after the second morning feed
1–1.30 p.m.	Provide a feed
	Expose to natural light
	Leisure time
2–3 p.m.	Within 1½–2 hours of waking, baby should be asleep again
	Read their sleep cues but don't allow them to stay awake longer than this suggested time frame
4–4.30 p.m.	Provide feed
	Expose to natural light
	Leisure time
5–6 p.m.	Asleep again within 1½–2 hours of waking
7–7.30 p.m.	Feed
7.30–11 p.m.	May nap on and off until your bedtime, with a last feed around 10–11 p.m., and feed then throughout the night as needed until morning
	Your baby's bedtime is quite late at the start but will get earlier as the first few months pass
	It is likely that you will keep your baby with you until then, sleeping on you or in a Moses basket or pram close to you until you go to bed
	Prepare for bed no more than 1½ hours after the last nap
	Take your baby to the bedroom and provide the night-time feed, and when you are ready, start using the percentage-of-wakefulness concept as your baby is going to sleep
	Provide night-time feeds, comfort and support as required
	Keep the night feed in the bedroom and be as non-disruptive as possible

Lucy Says

All babies are different and imposing a strict routine on your baby may not be appropriate. This is a guide and should be implemented with flexibility, keeping in mind your sleep-shaping approach and safe sleep, primarily ensuring that your child is responded to, getting enough to drink and gaining weight accordingly.

LUCY'S CHECKLIST

- ☑ Be very careful not to overstimulate or allow your baby to get overtired by staying awake too long. Some babies can only manage 45 minutes' wakefulness at the start of the day. This typically gets longer as the day goes on, with an hour and half to two hours' awake time at any one time. Always prepare for a nap 20 minutes before the end of the maximum wake period suggested.

- ☑ Spend time getting to know your baby – not every cry means they are hungry. Have a checklist: hungry, tired, cold, bored, nappy change, for example.

- ☑ Keep in mind that some babies need more assistance than others and really do need your help to sleep. Sleep ability skills may not become possible for another few months. In the interim, make sure that you facilitate the sleep process by observing all the other elements outlined.

- ☑ Beyond six weeks, start to create a consistent bedtime routine to set up the right sleep cues for baby. Understanding what happens next can make the transition from awake to asleep almost seamless for your baby.

- ☑ Focus on bedtime specifically, which will probably be quite late: work on putting your baby into bed relaxed but awake using the percentage-of-wakefulness concept. Stay nearby and soothe gently as they finish falling asleep. Physically comfort and support them as they develop the ability – if it doesn't feel right, then stop and try again at a later date.

Q *I am making great progress at bedtime, but the day sleep is impossible!*

It takes longer to establish daytime sleep, so napping can be disorganised until six months plus. Most babies benefit from three to eight naps of varied duration, within 45-minute to two-hour wake windows, throughout the day until bedtime and three-hourly feeds therein.

Many naps may still be short, about 20–45 minutes long, but will gradually lengthen as sleep matures and if they are getting enough sleep at the right time and learning to have an enhanced sleep ability. At the end of the month two, and ideally by the end of month three, you could probably start to phase out motion sleep in cars or swings for the first and maybe the second nap, and get them sleeping in the cot or sleeper, whatever you are using. The rest of the day sleeps can be motion-orientated thereafter.

Lucy Says

During the early months some babies will sleep better than others. All babies can become great sleepers in time and especially within the second half of the first year. Parents may find the early months draining and exhilarating at the same time, but don't worry. Longer stretches of sleep are just around the corner.

Feeding and sleeping suggestions: two to four months

Your baby's sleep is possibly becoming more mature and organised. You may see some longer stretches overnight, but don't worry if you are not. It is hard to manage, but all babies are different and by following my suggestions you will set a solid foundation for better sleep practices, ensuring that *your* baby reaches *their* optimum amount of sleep.

- Total amount of sleep: 10½–12 hours overnight with feeds
- Total amount of daytime sleep: four to five hours during the day

- Number of naps: three to six, depending on wake time and nap duration
- Daytime sleep will be becoming more organised with naps extending anything from 40 minutes to two to three hours per sleep segment
- Don't worry about nap amounts – get the balance between the naps working well and the duration will emerge in time
- Feeds: every three hours during the day, possibly longer overnight
- Night-time feeds may still be appropriate until closer to nine months

Q How often should I be feeding my baby?

I would anticipate that your feeding practice is now established and you are comfortably feeding more or less on a three-hourly basis through the day and possibly longer overnight if you are lucky! If your baby is still waking frequently overnight that is perfectly normal. Make sure you are observing all the other recommendations for your child's age range, then, as they get older, you can address night feeds as set out in Chapters 10 and 12. Your young baby will still require a number of night-time feeds until they start to get a bit older, and by six months onwards you may really see a pattern emerge.

Although I appreciate that it would be great if the night feeds diminished as early as possible, please understand that they may remain until at least nine months or so and we just have to meet that need.

Q I am really confused – what do you think about dream feeds?

As your baby gets older, bedtime starts to get earlier and you may be thinking about how best to manage the night-time feeds. There are many schools of thought on this. It can be helpful in times of sickness, and in Chapter 12 I discuss using a dream feed when trying to improve night sleep while retaining a feed, but I would not suggest it as an initial approach.

A dream or sleepy feed is where the parent initiates the night-time feed at a certain time —normally between 10 and 11.30 p.m. – when the child is still asleep. The baby is lifted and given a feed in the hopes that it will 'see them through' until morning. For some, this is effective and does exactly that so it is a worthwhile exercise for them.

However, I see a large number of babies who are being woken for a dream feed who then go on to wake frequently and additional feeds are provided. The feeds are possibly needed, but perhaps the dream feed is not, and the very act of initiating the feed is disrupting your child's inner rhythm and sleep, making the dream feed counter-productive.

I suggest a feed when your baby wakes, provided it is within a reasonable time of the last feed. This way it is baby-led and supported by you and there's a possibility of sleeping longer with parents moving towards reduced or no night-feed territory sooner – if your baby is biologically ready.

Q *I have heard that if I give my baby water when they wake up, then they will not be interested and will just stop waking*

I would *not* suggest cool boiled water as a milk-feed substitute. There is no rush to make your child sleep through when they still require a feed. Make all the other adjustments and the feeds will go away when your child is biologically able. If this does not emerge beyond nine months, then you can start observing a night-weaning exercise (see page 154) with GP consent.

From 2–4 months:

Wake time	6–7.30 a.m.	Start the day no later than 7.30 a.m. regardless of what has happened overnight
		Get out of bed and expose your baby to natural/bright light
		Provide a morning feed within the first 30 minutes of waking to anchor your day feeds, regardless of what feeds have happened overnight

Nap 1	7–9.30 a.m.	Prepare for your first nap within 1–2 hours of being awake Pay attention to your sleep baby's sleep cues and act on them If you don't see them looking tired, prepare for the nap 20 minutes before the end of the suggested wake period This nap may be as little as 40 minutes or it may be an hour or more Allow your baby to wake naturally, but wake them to maintain your next feed, which will be due three hours after the first morning feed
Awake	9–10.30 a.m.	Provide a feed within three hours of the morning feed. The timing will depend on the morning feed time Expose to natural light Leisure time
Nap 2	10.30 a.m.– 12.00 p.m.	Depending on time and duration of nap 1, prepare for the next nap within 1½–2 hours of being awake Don't plan your sleep time on the time that your baby has fed, you must base it on the time your baby woke and also read their sleep cues This nap may be as little as 40 minutes or it may be over an hour Allow your baby to wake naturally, but wake them to maintain your next feed, which will be due three hours after the second morning feed
Awake	1.30– 2.30 p.m.	Provide a feed within three hours of the last feed Expose to natural light Leisure time
Naps 3–5	3–4 p.m.	Depending on the time and duration of nap 2, provide a third/fourth/fifth nap as required within 1½–2 hours of being awake Your baby will then be awake from 4.30–6 p.m. at the latest and the next sleep will be bedtime, which will gradually get earlier to anywhere between 6 and 8 p.m., depending on when the last nap finishes

	4.30–5.30 p.m.	Provide a feed within three hours of the last one
		Consider a cluster or split feed so you can provide a feed closer to bedtime (see Lucy Says below)
	6.15–7.15 p.m.	Prepare for bed about 1¼–1½ hours after the final nap
		Provide the bath and/or bedtime routine
		Provide the bedtime feed or remainder of the last feed
		Operate the percentage-of-wakefulness approach
Sleep	6.30–8 p.m.	Within 1¼–1½ hours of the last nap, prepare for bedtime. Provide the remainder of the last feed and commence your bedtime routine, ideally using the percentage-of-wakefulness approach
Overnight	Till 6–7.30 a.m.	Your baby will still require night-time feed(s)
		Your baby may sleep for longer stretches, but still be wakeful in the later part of the night as you head towards morning
		Provide feeds accordingly and comfort and support as needed

Lucy Says

You may find that your breastfed baby is inclined to feed on and off throughout the evening. This is often referred to as cluster-feeding and is very typical. A split feed can be used for either a bottle or a breastfed baby, where you provide half the bottle or one side initially and then, within a short space of time, the rest of the feed and then put them to bed.

LUCY'S CHECKLIST

☑ During this time frame, night sleep may become more organised, and you can begin to concentrate on the quality and quantity of your child's sleep: the amount of sleep they get and the place that they sleep.

☑ There is a natural variation in how long babies in this age can sleep. Some will sleep more than others and, once again, this is not a failure on your part: it's just how they come.

☑ Feed in quiet places with few distractions so they can concentrate on the feed and satisfy their hunger.

☑ If you want your child to sleep in their sleeper/cot, then now try to avoid bringing them into your bed overnight. Return them to the cot after their night-time feed to avoid an expectation of bed-sharing if you can't or don't want to commit to that as a family.

☑ At the end of month three and ideally by the end of month four, you should probably phase out motion sleep in cars and swings for nap 1 and nap 2 and get them sleeping in the cot or sleeper, depending on what you are using. The rest of the day naps can be motion orientated.

☑ Be mindful of your baby's growth spurts and milestones, which can also disturb sleep. The Wonder Weeks app is a useful guide for checking whether that is the reason for any regressions.

☑ Towards the four-months mark, your baby is developing a better body clock and may be able to stay awake for longer periods, but you really need to avoid them getting overtired, fussy and hard to settle, as this will negatively impact the night-time sleep. Two hours of wakefulness is still a good guide.

☑ Neurologically the character of your baby's sleep is evolving and locking into place. Be mindful of sleep ability and what your baby associates with falling asleep, and try to allow them to perfect the skill of falling asleep at bedtime, with continued reduced parental input.

☑ If to date this task has been impossible, you may just need to resign yourself to it for a while longer and then from six months onwards begin to implement my effective stay-and-support approach.

Chapter 7

Four to Six Months: Sleep Regressions and Developmental Stages

Once you have survived the first few months you will ideally have a rhythm going, but don't panic if not. You can start to work on your child's sleep improvement at any time.

However, the period between four and six months is a bit of a no man's land for sleep – typically, it is too late to sleep shape and it is too early to implement sleep learning. Now, you may discover that you just need to tread water for the next few weeks, and then at six months, depending on the issues reported, you can start to create a formal plan. This doesn't mean that you cannot observe the feeding and sleeping suggestions for this age range – this alone can make a significant difference. I encourage you to do this, along with beginning the basis of a bedtime routine if you haven't already. But don't change 'how' you help your child to sleep currently – retain this for now and change from six months onwards with the stay-and-support approach.

Lucy Says

This timeframe and recommendation frustrates lots of parents and some decide to start the plan anyway. The results can be varied. Some will blaze a trail through the plan and use the stay-and-support approach with ease, and this obviously means that not only were you ready for change, but so was your child. Others will report all-out war, lots of unnecessary and unwanted crying and it may seem worse rather than better. My sterling recommendation is to wait to use the stay-and-support approach when your child is six months plus. That way then we know, in general, that they will be developmentally open to learning and that your efforts and theirs will achieve close to, if not all, your goals.

There is a lot going on developmentally between four and six months: it is undeniably tricky territory. It will be less tricky if you have been establishing the positive foundations as outlined in the previous chapters. But if you have not, then, along with the four-month regression (see below), you may find that your sleep is worse than ever, and there is little scope to make changes outside of the feeding and sleeping suggestions.

Don't despair! You can be preparing the scene, and although this may not seem helpful at the time, it often makes the learning cycle easier when you do go to address it at six months onwards.

Four-month regression

Q *My baby was sleeping great, just waking once a night for a feed, and now they're waking multiple times and I just don't know what to do*

For a lot of families, in the first few months sleep can be pretty good. You may have developed a rhythm to your day that seems to suit your child, and in return night-time sleep is reasonable, if not really good – only waking one or two times for a feed or actually sleeping overnight with little or no input from you. And then one day that all falls apart.

Welcome to the four-month regression. Or more accurately, welcome to sleep maturation. As mentioned previously, somewhere about four months sleep characteristically locks into place, and now what used to work because your baby's sleep was immature no longer works, as their brain has taken over the controls for sleep. Whatever they associate with going to sleep now needs to be repeated –and more in some cases – each time they cycle through sleep. This can be where feeding, rocking or holding 100 per cent to sleep may now start to work against you.

A higher level of adjustment can be required to help return to better sleep, rather than just waiting it out like some other developmental phases. The percentage-of-wakefulness approach may help with this phase, but not always.

Try not to worry. Your child is racing through neurodevelopmental stages. Their previously later bedtime biologically gets much earlier. They may be starting to show an interest in solid food. They will be learning that they exist independently to you. They may start to teethe or experience their first sickness. You may even be thinking about returning to work. It can be exceptionally challenging during this period, but with effort it can improve.

To help survive the four-month regression and four to six months period:

- Introduce my feeding and sleeping balances for this age range detailed below – pay particular attention to the wake time (this now becomes earlier: 6–7.30 a.m.), the suggested naptimes, nap durations and cut-off points for day sleep.
- Attempt the nap timings about 20 minutes before the suggested wake period so you are avoiding allowing your baby to become overtired.
- Encourage daytime sleep in any way that works for your child. If holding them keeps them asleep longer, commit to this.
- No naps after 5 p.m. – even if they only fell asleep at 4.45 p.m., ensure this nap ending to hormonally synchronise bedtime.
- Establish a bedtime routine in the bedroom that your child sleeps in.

- Implement the suggested bed timing only. Don't change your final milk feed or how you typically achieve sleep – continue with your usual strategies, but now aim with precision for your baby to be asleep for 7 p.m. (Whatever changes are required at bedtime will need to wait until 6 months so we know your baby is ready to learn via the stay-and-support approach.)
- Bring forward bedtime with immediate effect – there is no need to do this slowly: they are designed to go to sleep around 7 p.m.
- Create a dark environment for bedtime, overnight and naps – we need to strengthen sleep context now as much as possible.
- Share the load and draft in support during this time. It will pass, but you will need to work through this sensitively. That way, the sleep-learning exercise at six months plus will be easier for all.

Developmental stages

Your child will go through multiple developmental stages that may cause a sleep regression. The most notable is at four months, but there may be others too around eight to nine months, twelve to eighteen months and two years. It is not unusual for sleep to be affected by developmental achievements: they may routinely sleep well and then, without any symptoms of teething or sickness, you experience some uncharacteristic night-time activity. Growth spurts often overlap the developmental stages, but feed as needed and everything passes.

As a new skill is being learnt – rolling, pulling up to standing, walking or language – your child may stay awake for long periods of time practising their skill, and then, without need for your intervention, return to sleep. This tends to pass – most sleep regressions last for two to six weeks – but it can be extended when teething or sickness overlap. We need to be careful that we do not blame every sleep interruption on teething, sickness or leaps. They are only relevant if they accompany the symptoms outlined earlier.

Lucy Says

Any sleep interruption can be more challenging if your child does not routinely sleep well. If this particular stage overlaps with their current poor sleep practices, you may find that you need to support your child a lot overnight until this passes. Maybe you can also start to address the extra layer of issues with the help of this book.

What you *can* do is practise: give your child plenty of opportunity to develop the skill they are gaining. Make sure they practise this lots throughout the course of the day. Regardless of the skill, ensure that your child is getting lots of floor time and is free to roam, not spending too much time in a playpen, cordoned off in a small space in your living room or in the buggy, car seat or high chair. Do activities with them to help them get it out of their system, so they'll feel less like practising at bedtime and/or overnight. This won't stop it happening overnight, as that's where they will process everything they are learning, but it may reduce the vulnerabilities.

ROLLING

If rolling is their new skill, help your child become really good at going from back to front and over and again. The more efficient they become, the more capable they will be of getting comfortable overnight and not getting stuck. Now that they can roll – although you will continue to place on their back to sleep – you can let them assume a comfortable sleeping position, be that back, front or side. Don't keep putting your child on their side when they are going to sleep, as you run the risk that, when they move, they'll need you to 'rearrange' them all night long. Whatever position they assume, they need to be able to achieve it with your intervention.

Consider having them practise rolling in their sleeping bag, so they are also able to roll with the constraints of the bag. Master key words such as 'roll over' and poke their side gently with their finger to remind them what they can do, and repeat overnight as required.

Continue to observe safe sleep – it is important that there are no loose bedding items, and if to date you have been using a positioner or sleep aid such as a Sleepy Head, now is the time to retire these, as they typically do not support your child's current need to get comfortable in a larger space. A conventional cot now, over a sleeper crib, is a more suitable option. Before they needed a small, enclosed sleep environment; now they need space.

Lucy Says

At this stage, a swaddle is not appropriate. However, if you have been swaddling, I suggest a sleeping bag is the best way forward. There are a few schools of thought on this transition, but I like to introduce a sleeping bag by four months, allowing the arms free and letting your child figure out what to do with themselves without restraint. This takes time and they may need your support, but once they're rolling, arms-out is the safest, most appropriate option.

STANDING

If standing is the new skill (emerging from around 9 months onwards), then encourage plenty of practice by day too. Show them over and over again how to go from standing to sitting to lying down. Play games like ring-a-rosie – teach them the words that accompany the action: 'all fall down'. Show them in the cot how to go from standing to sitting by running their hand down the bars and underpin with the key words.

At bedtime or overnight you may need to stay with them to help them learn to lie down in the cot. Lie on the floor so that your body is lower than theirs. If you stand, kneel or sit on a chair, this will further encourage standing. When they first stand, allow them to get it out of their system. After a few minutes, lay them down once. If they stand up again, don't get into a power struggle or reinforce the behaviour – stay low on the floor yourself and encourage them down of their own accord. Even if they remain standing for a long time, try to wait them out so that they lie down themselves. If you stay low, they will be less inclined to stand anyway, as they will be attracted to being down at your level. If they get sleepy standing or sitting up, lay them down one more time.

CLIMBING

If they try to climb out of the cot, don't immediately rush to a big bed – a big-bed transition is more suitable for older children and generally not done as part of an effort to improve sleep. (In *The Baby Sleep Solution* I discuss 'in a bed too soon' in detail.) Supervise, if they try to climb – push their knee down and say 'no climbing'. Stay low on the floor and treat as above with standing.

A big bed is generally better introduced when your child routinely sleeps well, has finished daytime naps and is toilet-trained – see my Rule of Free: nap free, nappy free and over three!

Q *I don't normally stay when they are going to sleep – how should I handle this?*

If they have recently learnt to stand or climb then you may need to return to the cot-side to assist them through this stage. Once you feel they have accomplished this, either just start to leave again, provided they will allow you, or work through the stages to sleep detailed in Chapter 3.

Q *All of a sudden, my social baby is 'making strange'*

Separation anxiety is another developmental stage that peaks at various points as your child further develops separateness and self-awareness. It is most notable around four to six months, nine months, eighteen months and two years. It has an undermining effect on sleep, as sleep itself is a big separation, and this may make not staying with them at bedtime or being alone overnight a sensitive matter. As with the other developmental leaps, I encourage you to adopt certain practices by day to address the sensitivities at bedtime and night-time. Again, try not to allow each stage, leap and regression to stop you making progress. There are so many factors affecting positive sleep practices that waiting for each one to pass may mean that sleep is never addressed.

There are many activities you can do with your child that will help them to understand:

- Play disappearing-and-reappearing games like peek-a-boo, Jack-in-the-box and hiding items under blankets.
- Practise leaving your child in the living room while you go into the kitchen to get something – tell them you are going and return quickly so they understand you will come back.
- Don't sneak off on them if you are leaving the house. Always say goodbye, even if it upsets them – remember, we are building trust with them all the time.
- Whenever you play games designed to overcome or develop a skill, underpin with a key word or phrase –'wait', 'I'll be back' or 'here I am', for example. Then, when required, you can factor those words into your sleep practices too.
- Avoid holding your baby in arms all the time – make sure you are going down to them sometimes instead of always bringing them up to you.

Resisting one parent

My baby won't allow her dad to put her to bed – she only wants me and becomes hysterical if he attempts to do bedtime

This is a very common issue that can arise at any stage, and it can be an adverse reaction to either parent. I personally experienced this with my youngest child, Harry, who at eighteen months completely refused to let me do bedtime. The reasons for this are complex and, whatever the cause, we need to attempt to overcome it in a loving and mindful way.

One reason a baby might only want a particular parent is that they have certain associations for sleep with that parent. Take the breastfeeding mum, for example. If nursing is the only way your child can achieve their sleep, then the other parent attempting to do bedtime causes panic and an awareness of an inability to sleep without the breast – see more on this topic in Chapter 11.

One of my goals is that bedtime ultimately becomes interchangeable between parents. To establish this, a new way of going to sleep – using my stay-and-support approach (from six months) – often needs to be undertaken, so both parents have the same way of addressing sleep. To help with this, the timings provided – the bedtime number line (see page 133) – together with a formal bedtime routine in the bedroom with one parent is desirable. I always encourage the parent not breastfeeding to begin the new approach and to undertake bedtime on night 1 and night 2. I then introduce the other parent on night 3 and night 4. By making these changes, hopefully your baby will start to feel comfortable with both parents operating in a new way. If one parent comes in and takes over, we potentially undermine the parent–child relationship and inadvertently signal to them that the other parent is not trusted and they're not safe until rescued. So please be mindful about your actions when you start.

Include items in your bedtime routine to attract your child to bedtime with you. If a child is not breastfed, or hasn't been for a while, and prefers a certain parent at bedtime, I actually use that parent for bedtimes night 1 and night 2 and then introduce the less-preferred parent for nights 3 and 4. Don't be tempted to exclude the other parent for more than two bedtimes, as this can undermine our goal to establish interchangeability and disrupts continuity in the way the process unfolds.

I often reserve certain favourite or new toys or books for the less-preferred parent to attract the baby to them, but, more than that, it can be about the quality of time you spend with your child outside of sleep. I find resistance to a certain parent, when it has nothing to do with feeding, can actually be to do with the relationship by day. It is potentially your child's way of signalling their dissatisfaction with the amount of exclusive time you afford them. Easier said than done when you are working and/or there are more children in the household, but one of our tasks is to meet their continued needs, and time together is a significant one. Somehow, we need to make space for more exclusive connected time together. This does not include the bedtime routine or the time that you connect when feeding. It is entirely separate. Make a concerted effort to provide connected play – an undiluted concentration of time together with plenty of eye and physical contact. Colouring or reading doesn't always give us this, as we are side by side and not getting the necessary 'face time' for connection.

Ideally, we should spend 10–20 minutes of this deep and meaningful time with each child in the family unit at various points in the day. Work towards developing I-love-you rituals, games and activities that serve to deepen the quality of your relationship. Then you might find it easier to be allowed to take on bedtime. Joanna Fortune's *15 Minute Parenting* may be a good resource to help you here.

Q *I have tried this but my child just won't allow Mum to do bedtime – I find this very upsetting*

Sometimes, the child's need to have a particular parent undertake bedtime is so strong for them that trying to reverse this is too distressing. This is not a reflection on you or your parenting. If you have attempted to reverse this and they are not willing participants, you may need to temporarily pick your battles and allow one parent to continue bedtime for the foreseeable future. You can continue to make all the other changes required based on your situation.

In the background, the less-preferred parent can continue to strengthen the bonds between them and try again at a later date, when your child may be more open to this dynamic.

While it is important to encourage interchangeability, the task or attempt is never more important than the actual relationship with your child. There is a season and a reason for many tendencies, and while we can do our best to provide fertile ground, unless they are entirely immersed in our plans, we must ensure that the relationship is lovingly intact at all times.

Lucy Says

Solid food introduction is recommended by six months. Some of you, under your GP's supervision, will commence this practice sooner for a variety of reasons, e.g. reflux. But I would caution against early solid-food introduction in an effort to improve sleep as there is no evidence to support this – in fact, some studies have shown that it can make sleep worse! Plenty of appropriate information is available for parents beginning this journey. Speak with your GP or health visitor and see also what expert registered dietician Caroline O'Connor has to say in Chapter 15.

Feeding and sleeping suggestions: four to six months

- Total amount of night-time sleep: 10–12 hours with or without feed(s), depending on the child
- Total amount of daytime sleep: three to four hours
- Number of naps: three to five
- Feeds: three to four hourly, with or without solid food as appropriate
- Suggested milk need: 1,035ml in a 24-hour period and/or breastfeeds

Wake time	6–7.30 a.m.	Wake up by 7.30 a.m. to regulate the body clock, regardless of what has happened overnight Feed and/or breakfast, if established and age appropriate
Nap 1	8–9.30 a.m.	This nap should start within 1½–2 hours of waking Can be 45 minutes to 1 hour in duration Allow to wake naturally or waken after 1½ hours maximum

Awake/ leisure time	10–11.30 a.m.	Timing of the second feed and lunch, if established, will depend on wake time and nap duration
		There is a 1½–2 hour window of wakefulness before nap 2
		Feed and/or lunch should be over in time for the nap
Nap 2	11 a.m.– 12.30 p.m.	Child should be put down within 1½–2 hours of waking from nap 1
		Pay attention to sleep signals
		Nap 2 should ideally be an hour or more
		Allow your child to wake naturally or wake them to keep your next feed time in place
Awake/ leisure time	2–3 p.m.	Feed on wake-up
Nap 3–5	3–4 p.m.	Depending on the time and duration of second nap, provide further naps within 1½–2 hours of waking from each one
		Can be 10 minutes to an hour in duration
		These naps can be on the go in the car or buggy, not the cot, as it can be too difficult for most babies
		Wake by 4.30–5 p.m. at the latest
	5–5.30 p.m.	Dinner time, with protein and carbohydrate, if age appropriate and established
	6–6.15 p.m.	Bedtime feed
		This should be away from the bedroom with the lights on – nothing to do with sleep
	6.20–6.30 p.m.	Start bath, if doing one, and/or the bedtime routine in the bedroom where your child will sleep
	6.50 p.m.	Place your child into the cot
		Use the percentage-of-wakefulness approach or your usual strategy to enable them to sleep
Sleep	7 p.m.	Aim for your child to be asleep, maintaining a two-hour window of wakefulness between the end of the last nap and being in bed asleep

Chapter 8

Sleeping Through the Night

Q *How do I get my child to sleep through the night?*

This is the most commonly asked question. Regretfully, there is no magic formula, silver bullet or golden nugget. It is a combination of elements:

- Understanding
- Information
- Adjustments
- Changes
- Hard work
- Patience

My suggestions are designed to continually move you closer to this tendency, but we need to be informed and manage our expectations as parents. Rather than aiming for sleeping through the night, aim for more consolidated, less interrupted, deeper sleep with reduced parental input, when developmentally and age relevant for your child. This way you are not setting yourself up for feeling like you have failed if your baby doesn't sleep as well as your friend's or your sister's baby – every child really is different.

In earlier chapters, I have discussed the typical barriers to better sleep. In *The Baby Sleep Solution*, I outline in great detail a plan you can create to arrive at your goals. This book is about easily digestible pieces of information that address the regular queries I receive about strengthening a child's relationship with sleep.

To move closer to better overnight sleep, the following generally need to be established:

- ☑ Age relevance
- ☑ Age-appropriate feeding and sleeping balances
- ☑ Required changes at bedtime
- ☑ Overnight plan
- ☑ Predictable responses

Age relevance

Before six months, while some children can sleep incredibly well, many do not. I believe that it is not until at least six months that you can begin refining the adjustments that you have made to date, if any. If until now you have been winging it, then you can begin to make adjustments to move you towards sleeping better.

Lucy Says

Even after six months of age, although sleep ability is more apparent, your unique child's ability is exactly that – unique to them, in how they perceive the world and how you respond to them.

So your child needs to be at least six months old for you to think about achieving more, better, deeper sleep, if it hasn't emerged yet on its own or with the changes you have made to date. After six months, it is all to play for.

Age-appropriate feeding and sleeping balances

If we have not already, we now need to apply the timings with accuracy. Better sleep is achieved with regular wake times, exposure to bright and natural light during wake times, naps attempted before your child becomes overtired and a synchronicity between naps. So make sure the suggested fixed feed, nap-gap dynamic and bedtime number line are observed as outlined, with precision.

It can sound very prescriptive, but it is very effective.

Q *I have done everything you suggest and it is not working*

I know from experience that, outside of underlying medical issues, weak spots can be created by parents within the guidance. These are, typically:

- Not observing the morning wake time together with/or the timings suggested for nap 1
- Not waking on nap 1 as suggested
- Not observing the solid- or fixed-feed recommendations
- Selecting a later bedtime that suits you better
- Not entirely addressing night-time activity

Even a small change to my recommendations might undermine your effort. My timing suggestions are based on the science of sleep – they ensure that sleep is achieved in sync with the natural body clock and this, with all the other suggestions, helps to encourage sleeping better through the night.

Observe the timing that fits your child's age today. However, if they were born prematurely, work from their corrected age instead. Commit to the plan for three to four weeks and underpin with the stay-and-support approach as needed. You will start to see your sleep goals emerge, but not without additional challenges as you proceed.

Changes at bedtime

What happens at bedtime can decide the course of overnight and daytime sleep. Although we can feel that bedtime is easy and the best part of our child's sleep, often how bedtime is approached is the cause (although not obvious) of the issues reported. Chapter 11 addresses common bedtime issues that occur and can undermine progress, but in the meantime bear this mind:

- Whatever your child associates with falling asleep at bedtime – a bottle, a breastfeed, a rub, tuck or rock, music, white noise, a kiss on the forehead – may leave you vulnerable to unnecessary or unwanted night-time activity.
- Your child requires a high-level sleep ability at bedtime specifically for a high-level or complete sleep ability to emerge, with your support, overnight and into the daytime too.
- Making all the suggested changes but keeping your typical approach at bedtime is often the barrier to sleep success. There is merit and method, reason and consequence to all of the recommendations that I make.
- The concept of the fixed feed is important to ensure no partial dependency exists in this capacity.
- Going à la carte on the suggestions may diminish the efficacy of the plan.

Overnight approach

When you are attempting to improve the overnight period, then whatever your child typically expects from you – be it night feeds, bed-sharing, rocking and so on – is replaced with the techniques outlined in the stay-and-support approach discussed in Chapter 3. Use this at bedtime as required and into the overnight period too. Addressing the timings and changing how you operate at bedtime will not magically correct your overnight sleep. Try to think of sleep in segments:

- Bedtime
- Overnight
- Early morning
- Nap

Each sleep segment is related but also a separate entity, and each sleep segment needs attention to enhance the next sleep segment. Each sleep segment can have either a positive or negative effect on the next. Some families will make small adjustments on one sleep segment and that change alone *does* unlock sleep ability, but the majority of us will need to work on each sleep segment individually as part of the process.

Predictable responses

The stay-and-support approach replaces your original tendencies at bedtime, if required, and certainly for overnight and naps. It takes time, patience and commitment on your part and learning and understanding on your child's.

The overnight and early morning sleep segments can be the hardest to work on and, depending on your child's age and stage, it can take three to four weeks *plus* to see improvements emerging – but they will. This is a process and it moves along with your help. Naps start initially based on the wake-window timings and then graduate to clock-based timings, so you will need to keep adjusting and reviewing what needs to change and be worked on.

When I am working directly with a family, with all the knowledge at my fingertips, it can take this length of time. So on your own, with the book(s), it may take longer – but keep assessing for improvement, and provided you are comfortable with your efforts and it feels right, then continue, as your hard work *will* produce a yield.

As you work through the phases and stages, and episodes of teething or sickness, it's important that you respond consistently when addressing your child's sleep, as unfortunately, due to the behavioural component of sleep, a varied response may give you a varied result. Although challenging, sticking to what you have decided will be key to your sleep-learning outcome.

Lucy Says

Once you get started, then the process of learning is often represented by

- The bedtime sleep segment improving with the new approach within a few days
- The overnight sleep segment improving over 10–21 nights, depending on the decisions you have made, your consistency, your child's age, how long the issues have been occurring and so on
- The early morning sleep segment taking two to six weeks to overcome
- Going for naps starting to get easier, taking 10–21 days to improve too

---

When I am asked how to help a child sleep through the night, you can see now, given the many factors involved, that there is not just one answer or solution.

I like to address the sleep segments in a round, starting with bedtime then on to the other sleep segments, more or less in one go. Although this can feel daunting, it seems to work well. On the day you plan to start, ideally, follow the timings but still achieve day sleep as before, then, starting with bedtime, introduce the new approach. For example, start with bedtime on Friday night, observe the approach overnight and begin the same approach with naps on Saturday morning.

If you are struggling with certain areas, understand that whatever time, effort and pain you endure now is an investment in your child's sleep forevermore. That is a good return, I would say!

> *'All I can say is that this approach changed our lives. Honestly, if my son can learn anyone can! He was an awful sleeper from day one. Only napped on me or my husband, would never sleep for more than two to three hours at night and then was up every 40–60 minutes for the rest of the night until 3 a.m. when the only way to get him to sleep was to let him sleep on us ... which meant we were on shifts to do this for him. I was a shell of myself and had zero time for my three-year-old daughter. It has taken a month to really understand the routines and advice and implement them, and also, more importantly, even though it killed me to wait to try the book, six months plus is a great age to start. Before this I wanted it so badly but I knew he was too young and just wouldn't take to it, which would make me feel like a failure and make the whole process unnecessarily long. Every baby is different and Lucy's method acknowledges that. But there are some fundamental biological truths about humans and sleep and routine and feeding that do apply across the board. Like I've said, if my little man can go from probably five hours of broken sleep a night and only napping on us to sleeping two 90-minute naps in his cot and from 7 p.m.–6.30 a.m. at night, then anyone can!'*
>
> *– Helen, GP and mum of two*

Chapter 9

Routines

As you know now, biological timekeeping and overtiredness make up a significant portion of the sleep challenges that parents experience. In my first book, I looked at establishing an age-relevant feeding and sleeping balance to the day. I am including this information here too, with some adjustments, informed by the issues parents often have when making these sleep improvements.

Under 18 months of age, there are two dimensions of timings:

- Phase 1 – wake-window timings: these are based on an age-appropriate wake period (how long your child can stay awake for) and allow you to establish napping ability (see Chapter 14).

- Phase 2 – clock-based timings: once your child is starting to sleep better, to further futureproof your sleep, we calibrate the day by basing our timings on the clock rather than intervals of time. (If you need more help in establishing the day's layout, refer to *The Baby Sleep Solution* and Chapter 14 in this book.)

Feeding and sleeping suggestions: six to eight months

PHASE 1: WAKE-WINDOW TIMINGS

- Total amount of night-time sleep: 10–12 hours with or without a feed, depending on the child
- Night-time feeds may still be appropriate until closer to nine months
- Total amount of daytime sleep: three to three and a half hours
- Number of naps: three to four
- Feeds: four hourly, with solid food as appropriate
- Suggested milk need six–seven months: 700–960ml
- Suggested milk need seven–eight months: 420–630ml

Wake time First feed Breakfast	6–7.30 a.m.	From 6 a.m. and no later than 7.30 a.m., get up and start the day
		Provide the first milk feed within the first half hour and breakfast within the next half hour
		Wake your child by 7.30 a.m. if still asleep to regulate the body clock regardless of what has happened overnight
Nap 1 – cot	8–9.30 a.m. (avoid naps commencing before 7.40 a.m.)	This nap should start within 2 hours of waking
		Prepare for this nap 1 hour 40 minutes after getting up
		This nap can be 45 minutes to an hour long
		Allow to wake naturally or waken after 1½ hours

Awake/ leisure/ connected time Second feed Lunch	10 a.m.– 11.30	Between nap 1 and nap 2 provide the second milk feed and lunch The time will depend on wake time and nap duration There is a 2–3 hour window of wakefulness after nap 1 ends and nap 2 begins Feed and lunch should be over in time for the nap even if it seems really early – we will adjust this in time Around seven months onwards this milk feed is often replaced with the introduction of meat protein
Nap 2 – cot	11–12.30 p.m.	Start time of nap 2 depends on nap 1's start time and duration Your child should be put down within 2–3 hours of waking from nap 1. Prepare for this nap initially 1 hour and 40 minutes after waking from nap 1, then extend to 2 hours and 10 minutes after within week 1, and 2 hours and 40 minutes by week 2 Nap 2 will ideally be 1 hour+ in duration Allow to wake naturally or wake to keep your next feed in place
Awake/ leisure/ connected time Third feed/ snack	2–3.30 p.m.	Milk feed/healthy snack, depending on last feed time
Nap 3 – car/buggy	3–4 p.m.	Depending on time and duration of nap 2, provide a third nap as needed within 1½–2½ hours of waking Nap 3 can be 10 minutes to 1 hour in duration Wake by 5 p.m. at the latest This nap can be on the go in the car, buggy or sling – not the cot as this can be too challenging for most babies Observe the bedtime number line and the nap-gap dynamic

Dinner time	5–5.30 p.m.	Provide dinner, with carbohydrate and meat protein, when established
Fixed feed	5.45–6 p.m.	Provide bedtime milk feed Do this away from the bedroom with the lights on, so that it has nothing to do with sleep Remove the feed by 6.15 p.m., regardless of intake, to ensure at least 45 minutes between end of feed and sleep time
Bedtime routine	6.20–6.30 p.m.	Start bath and/or bedtime routine in the bedroom where your child will sleep With or without a bath, the routine must start by 6.30 p.m.
Into cot	6.50 p.m.	Place your child into the cot Use the stay-and-support approach as required
Aim to be asleep	7 p.m.	Aim for your child to be asleep, observing no more than a 2–2½ hour window of wakefulness between the end of the last nap and being in bed asleep

You may need a fourth nap if the first three naps are short and thus day sleep is ending too early. In that case, provide a fourth nap to allow day sleep to finish as close to 5 p.m. as possible. If you can't manage a third or fourth nap or naps are finished early (before 3–4 p.m.), you may need to bring bedtime forward to 6 p.m. onwards, adjusting everything by one hour or the corresponding amount. This is not a long-term strategy but it's a good short-term one as you work on the issues and attempt to stop the overtired cycle from spiralling.

PHASE 2: CLOCK-BASED TIMINGS

As your child's sleep starts to improve, you often find yourself in an early cycle – early waking means early naps, which means day sleep is routinely finished too early, resulting in either a too long nap-gap dynamic or an early bedtime that can further fuel the cycle.

Once you have been actively working on this for ten days, bedtime and naps are getting easier and you are managing to move further away from the cot, then I suggest making the following changes.

Nap 1 – cot	9–10 a.m. (avoid naps commencing before 9 a.m.)	We no longer work on the wake period, unless your child is waking from around 7 a.m. onwards If not, start to move the first nap from 8 a.m. by five minutes every day – without going backwards – so that within the next week or so this nap routinely begins no earlier than 9 a.m., despite waking early This nap can be 45 minutes to over an hour in duration Allow to wake naturally or waken after 1½ hours
Awake/leisure/ connected time Second feed Lunch	10 a.m.–1.30 p.m.	Between nap 1 and nap 2 provide the second milk feed and lunch The time will depend on wake time and nap duration There is a 2–3 hour window of wakefulness after nap 1 ends and nap 2 begins Feed and lunch should be over in time for the nap even if it seems really early – we will adjust this in time Around seven months onwards this milk feed is often replaced with the introduction of meat protein

Nap 2 – cot	11 a.m.–1.30 pm	Start time of nap 2 depends on nap 1's start time and duration
		Your child should be put down within 2–3 hours of waking from nap 1, slowly extending this wake period
		Prepare for this nap initially 1 hour and 40 minutes after waking from nap 1, then extend to 2 hours and 10 minutes within week 1 and 2 hours and 40 minutes by week 2
		Nap 2 will ideally be 1 hour+ in duration
		Allow to wake naturally or wake to keep your next feed in place
		As your baby gets closer to eight months, nap 2 needs to start around 1–1.30 p.m. so that when nap 3 is retired at eight months+ the nap-gap dynamic is observed
Awake/leisure/connected time Third feed and snack	2–3.30 p.m.	Milk feed/healthy snack, depending on last feed time
Nap 3 – car/buggy	3–4 p.m.	Depending on the time and duration of nap 2, provide a third nap within 1½–2½ hours of waking
		Nap 3 can be 10 minutes to 1 hour in duration
		Waken by 4.30–5 p.m. at the latest
		This nap can be on the go in the car, buggy or sling – not the cot, as it can be too challenging for most babies
		As this nap starts to go, adjust nap 2 as above
		Continue to apply the bedtime number line (page 133) and the age-relevant nap-gap dynamic (page 174) to underpin your efforts to date.

Feeding and sleeping suggestions: eight to twelve months

PHASE 1: WAKE-WINDOW TIMINGS

- Total amount of night-time sleep: 10½–12 hours
- From 9 months+ (or before): night feeds generally not required
- Total amount of daytime sleep: 2½–3 hours
- Number of naps: two to three
- Feeds: three milk feeds, 420–630ml, and/or breastfeeds with solid food as appropriate

Wake time First feed Breakfast	6–7.30 a.m.	From 6 a.m. and no later than 7.30 a.m., get up and start the day
		Provide the first milk feed within the first half hour and breakfast within the next half hour
		Wake your child by 7.30 a.m. if still asleep to regulate the body clock regardless of what has happened overnight
Nap 1 – cot	8–9.30 a.m.	This nap should start within two hours of waking
		Prepare for this nap 1 hour and 40 minutes after getting up
		Begin your naptime routine within 1 hour and 40 minutes of getting up
		This nap can be 45 minutes to 1 hour+ in duration
		Allow to wake naturally or waken after 1½ hours

Awake/ leisure/ connected time Lunch	10–11.30 a.m.	Between nap 1 and nap 2 provide lunch with water This timing will depend on wake time and nap duration There is a 3-hour window of wakefulness after nap 1 ends and nap 2 begins Lunch should be over in time for the nap even if it seems really early – we will adjust it in time
Nap 2 – cot	11 a.m.–1.30 p.m.	Start time of nap 2 depends on nap 1 start time and duration Begin your naptime routine within 2 hours and 40 minutes of waking from nap 1 Your child should be put down within 3 hours of waking from nap 1 Nap 2 will ideally be 1 hour+ in duration Allow to wake naturally or waken by 3.30 p.m. at the latest
Awake/ leisure/ connected time Second feed and snack	2–3.30 p.m.	Milk feed/healthy snack depending on last feed time
Possible back-up nap	3–4 p.m.	Your child may need a third nap starting between 3–4 p.m. if they haven't had enough sleep in the day or if your naps are finishing too early. This should be a motion sleep Awake by 4.30 p.m. at the latest and bedtime stays the same If naps have been short or finished too early (2–2.30 p.m.) and you can't manage a back-up nap, you will need to bring bedtime forward to 6 p.m. by adjusting dinner and last feed and start of bedtime routine by 1 hour Observe the bedtime number line and the nap-gap dynamic

Dinner time	5–5.30 p.m.	Provide dinner with carbohydrate and meat protein when established
Fixed feed	5.45–6 p.m.	Provide bedtime milk feed Do this away from the bedroom with the lights on, so that it has nothing to do with sleep Remove the feed by 6.15 p.m., regardless of intake, to ensure at least 45 minutes between end of feed and sleep time
Bedtime routine	6.20–6.30 p.m.	Start bath and/or bedtime routine in the bedroom where your child will sleep With or without a bath, the routine must start by 6.30 p.m.
Into cot	6.50 p.m.	Place your child into the cot Use stay-and-support approach as required
Aim to be asleep	7 p.m.	Aim for your child to be asleep by 7 p.m., observing not more than a 3–4 hour window of wakefulness between the end of the last nap and being in bed asleep If the final nap is finished early, bring forward bedtime to accommodate this

PHASE 2: CLOCK-BASED TIMINGS

As your child's sleep starts to improve, you often find yourself in an early cycle – early waking means early naps, which means day sleep is routinely finished too early, resulting in either a too long nap-gap dynamic or an early bedtime that can further fuel the cycle.

Once you have been actively working on this for ten days, bedtime and naps are getting easier and you are managing to move further away from the cot, then I suggest making the following changes.

Nap 1 – cot	9–10 a.m. (avoid naps commencing before 9 a.m.)	We no longer work on the wake period unless your child is waking from around 7 a.m. If not, start to move the first nap from 8 a.m. by five minutes every day – without going backwards – so that within the next week or so this nap routinely begins no earlier than 9 a.m., despite waking early This nap can be min 45 minutes to 1 hour+ in duration Allow to wake naturally or waken after 1½ hours
Awake/ leisure/ connected time Second feed, if appropriate Lunch	10 a.m.–1.30 p.m.	Between the first and second nap provide the second milk feed, if appropriate, and lunch The time will depend on wake time and nap duration There is a 2–3 hour window of wakefulness after nap 1 ends and nap 2 begins Feed and lunch should be over in time for the nap even if it seems really early – we will adjust this in time Around seven months onwards this milk feed is often replaced with the introduction of meat protein
Nap 2 – cot	1.30 p.m.	Ideally, this should not start before 1.30 p.m. Your child should be put down within 3 hours of waking from nap 1 Allow to wake naturally or waken by 3.30 p.m.
Awake/ leisure/ connected time Third feed and snack	2.30–3.30 p.m.	Milk feed/healthy snack depending on last feed time

Back-up nap while naps are finishing too early		Depending on time and duration of second nap, provide a third nap within 2½ hours of waking from nap 2
		Nap 3 can be 10 minutes to 1 hour in duration
		Waken by 4.30 p.m.at the latest
		This nap can be on the go in the car, buggy or sling – not the cot, as this can be too challenging for most babies
		This nap will retire as your child is getting more rest by day and nap 2 is adjusted later
		Continue to apply the bedtime number line (page 133) and the age-relevant nap-gap dynamic (page 174) to underpin your efforts to date

Feeding and sleeping suggestions: twelve to eighteen months

PHASE 1: WAKE-WINDOW TIMINGS

- Total amount of night-time sleep: 10½–12 hours
- From 9 months (or before): night feeds are generally not required
- Total amount of daytime sleep: 2–2½ hours
- Number of naps: two to three
- Feeds: two to three milk feeds, 240–420ml, and/or breastfeeds with solid food as appropriate

Wake time First feed Breakfast	6–7.30 a.m.	From 6 a.m. and no later than 7.30 a.m., get up and start the day
		Provide the first milk feed within the first half hour and breakfast within the next half hour
		Wake your child by 7.30 a.m. if still asleep to regulate the body clock regard-less of what has happened overnight

Nap 1 – cot	8–9.30 a.m. (avoid naps commencing before 7.40 a.m.)	This nap should start within 2–3 hours of waking Begin naptime routine 2 hours and 10 minutes after getting up – extend this to 2 hours and 40 minutes if they resist sleep after the first few days This nap can be at least 45 minutes to 1 hour+ in duration Allow to wake naturally or waken after 1½ hours – this may need to be limited to 1 hour if nap 2 is increasingly hard to achieve
Awake/ leisure/ connected time Lunch	10–11.30 a.m.	Between nap 1 and nap 2 provide lunch with water This timing will depend on wake time and nap duration There is a 3-hour window of wakefulness after nap 1 ends and nap 2 begins Lunch should be over in time for the nap even if it seems really early – we will adjust it in time
Nap 2 – cot	11 a.m.– 1.30 p.m.	Start time of nap 2 depends on nap 1 start time and duration Begin naptime routine 2 hours and 40 minutes after waking from nap 1 Your child should be put down within 3 hours of waking from nap 1 Nap 2 will ideally be 1 hour+ in duration Allow to wake naturally or waken by 3.30 p.m. at the latest
Awake/ leisure/ connected time Second feed and snack	2–3.30 p.m.	Milk feed/healthy snack depending on last feed time

Possible back-up nap	3–4 p.m.	Your child may need a third nap starting between 3 and 4 p.m. if they haven't had enough sleep in the day or if your naps are finishing too early. This should be a motion sleep
		Awake by 4.30 p.m. at the latest and bedtime stays the same
		If naps have been short or finished too early (by 2–2.30 p.m.) and you can't manage a back-up nap, you will need to bring bedtime forward to 6 p.m. by adjusting dinner and last feed and start of bedtime routine by 1 hour
		Observe the bedtime number line and the nap-gap dynamic
Dinner time	5–5.30 p.m.	Provide dinner with carbohydrate and meat protein when established
Fixed feed	5.45–6 p.m.	Provide bedtime milk feed
		Do this away from the bedroom with the lights on, so that it has nothing to do with sleep
		Remove the feed by 6.15 p.m., regardless of intake, to ensure at least 45 minutes between end of feed and sleep time
Bedtime routine	6.20–6.30 p.m.	Start bath and/or bedtime routine in the bedroom where your child will sleep
		With or without a bath, the routine must start by 6.30 p.m.
Into cot	6.50 p.m.	Place your child into the cot
		Use stay-and-support approach as required
Aim to be asleep	7 p.m.	Aim for your child to be asleep by 7 p.m., observing not more than a 3–4 hour window of wakefulness between the end of the last nap and being in bed asleep
		If the final nap is finished early, bring forward bedtime to accommodate this

PHASE 2: CLOCK-BASED TIMINGS

As your child's sleep starts to improve, you often find yourself in an early cycle – early waking means early naps, which means day sleep is routinely finished too early, resulting in either a too long nap-gap dynamic or an early bedtime that can further fuel the cycle.

Once you have been actively working on this for ten days, bedtime and naps are getting easier and you are managing to move further away from the cot, then I suggest making the following changes.

Nap 1 – cot	9–10 a.m. (avoid naps commencing before 9 a.m.)	We no longer work on the wake period unless your child is waking from around 7 a.m. If not, start to move the first nap from 8 a.m. by five minutes every day – without going backwards – so that within the next week or so this nap routinely begins no earlier than 9 a.m., despite waking early This nap can be min 45 minutes to 1 hour+ in duration Allow to wake naturally or waken after 1½ hours
Awake/leisure/ connected time Second feed (if appropriate) Lunch	10 a.m.–1.30 p.m.	Between the first and second nap provide a mid-morning snack and lunch as appropriate There is a 3-hour wake window between the end of nap 1 and when nap 2 should begin Lunch is provided before this nap so that they go into it on a full stomach
Nap 2 – cot	1.30 p.m.	Ideally, don't start before 1.30 p.m. Your child should be put down within 3 hours of waking from nap 1 Allow to wake naturally or waken by 3.30 p.m. at the latest

Awake/leisure/ connected time Second feed and snack	2.30–3.30 p.m.	Milk feed/healthy snack depending on last feed time
Possible back-up nap while naps are still finishing too early – may need to adjust bedtime forward while the gap is closing		Depending on time and duration of second nap, provide a third nap as required within 2½ hours of waking from nap 2 Nap 3 can be 10 minutes to 1 hour in duration Waken by 4.30 p.m. at the latest This nap can be on the go in the car, buggy or sling – not the cot as this can be too challenging for most babies This nap will retire as your child is getting more rest by day and nap 2 is adjusted later
		Continue to apply the bedtime number line (see page 133) and the age-relevant nap-gap dynamic (see page 174) to underpin your efforts to date

Feeding and sleeping suggestions: eighteen months to two-and-a-half years

- Total amount of night-time sleep: 10½–12 hours
- Night-time feeds: generally not required – if in doubt discuss with your GP
- Total amount of daytime sleep: 1–2 hours+
- Number of naps: one to two
- Feeds: 150–210ml per day and/or breastfeeds with three solid meals and two to three snacks as appropriate

When your child is ready for one nap a day, then the single nap ideally starts as late as possible so it covers the day and protects the nap-gap dynamic and avoids early waking. A single nap that starts too early, although long enough and although bedtime is age appropriate, often creates too long a wake period before bedtime, which increases your vulnerability to unwanted and unnecessary night-time activity.

A single nap ideally starts around 1 p.m., so try to move to this time with immediate effect, delaying and distracting as necessary. If they cannot cope beyond 11.30 a.m. then move the single nap out by 15 minutes every two days or so, so the nap can start closer to 1 p.m. or beyond. If they can't get beyond 10 a.m. due to early waking, then provide the filler nap as outlined in the table below.

Wake time First feed Breakfast	6–7.30 a.m.	From 6 a.m. and no later than 7.30 a.m., get up and start the day
		Provide the first milk feed within the first half hour and breakfast within the next half hour
		Wake your child no later than 7.30 a.m. if still asleep to regulate the body clock regardless of what has happened overnight
Filler nap, if very tired before 10 a.m. – car/ buggy/ couch	9–10 a.m. (avoid naps commencing before 9 a.m.)	If your child is waking very early and is super-tired then provide a filler nap
		This nap should start within 3 hours of waking
		Provide this nap in the car or buggy or on the couch and wake your child after 20–30 minutes – it is just to help you position the main nap as late as possible
Awake/leisure/ connected time Lunch	11.30 a.m.– 12.30 p.m.	Have high-level activity (e.g. playground, walk, soft-play centre) in the morning
		Provide lunch with water
		Lunch should be over in time for the nap so they go into the nap on a full stomach

Main nap – cot	12.30 –1 p.m.	Start the main nap ideally from 1 p.m. onwards
		If you need a filler nap, as above, then prepare for the main nap 2 hours and 40 minutes after waking them, but a single nap starting around 1 p.m. is preferable to underpin the nap-gap dynamic and bedtime
		This nap will ideally be 1–2 hours+ in duration
		Allow them to wake naturally or waken by 3.30 p.m. at the latest
		If this starts to interfere with bedtime then wake by 3 p.m. and review
Feed and snack Activity	2–3.30 p.m.	Milk feed and healthy snack High-level activity Observe the bedtime number line and the nap-gap dynamic
Dinner time	5–5.30 p.m.	Provide dinner with carbohydrate and meat protein when established
Fixed feed	5.45–6 p.m.	Provide bedtime milk feed
		Do this away from the bedroom with the lights on, so that it has nothing to do with sleep
		Remove by 6.15 p.m., regardless of intake, to ensure at least 45 minutes between end of feed and sleep time
Bedtime routine	6.20–6.30 p.m.	Start bath (if doing one) and/or the bedtime routine in the bedroom where your child will sleep
		With or without a bath the routine must start by 6.30 p.m.

Into cot	6.50 p.m.	Place your child into the cot
		Use stay-and-support approach as required
Aim to be asleep	7 p.m.	Aim for your child to be asleep by 7 p.m., observing not more than a 4–5 hour window of wakefulness between the end of the last nap and being in bed asleep
		If the final nap is finished early (before 2–2.30 p.m.) bring forward bedtime to accommodate this
		Initially aim for 7 p.m. but as your child gets better rested and a later bedtime emerges, start to prepare for bedtime 45 minutes before this time

If your child routinely falls asleep later, you can start to adjust bedtime as follows.

	For a natural bedtime of 7.30 p.m.	For a natural bedtime of 8 p.m.
Bedtime routine	6.50 p.m.	7.20 p.m.
Into cot	7.10 p.m.	7.40 p.m.
Aim to be asleep	7.30 p.m.	8 p.m.

Feeding and sleeping suggestions: two-and-a-half to six years

- Total amount of night-time sleep: 10½–12 hours
- Night-time feeds: generally not required – if in doubt discuss with your GP
- Total amount of daytime sleep: 0–2 hours+
- Number of naps: zero to one
- Feeds: 150–210ml per day and/or breastfeeds with three solid meals and two to three snacks as appropriate

The daytime sleep need will usually be in the region of 0–2 hours, with most children up to three years on one nap per day and beyond three either shrinking their nap or not napping every day as they work towards no nap somewhere between three and four years of age.

When still napping, the nap needs to start closer to 12.30–1 p.m. to create the right balance. If your current nap is earlier than this, either adjust it with immediate effect, or adjust it gradually by moving it by 15 minutes every two days until the naps begins closer to 12.30–1 p.m. Don't be concerned with the wake period between getting up and the nap – it is the wake period between the nap and bedtime that has pernicious implications if too long. Limit this nap to 3 p.m. initially and 2.30 p.m. if it starts to affect bedtime.

When your child is no longer napping, provide 'quiet time' – ideally, reading, listening to music or audiobooks, but not television or electronic media – for about an hour around the time the nap should happen.

Wake time	6–7.30 a.m.	From 6 a.m. and no later than 7.30 a.m., get up and start the day
		Provide drink within the first half hour and breakfast within the next half hour
		Wake your child by 7.30 a.m. if still asleep to regulate their body clock, regardless of what has happened overnight
Leisure Lunch	11.30 a.m.– 12.00 p.m.	Have high-level activity in the morning time and provide lunch with water
		Make sure lunch is provided before the nap (if applicable) so your child goes into the nap on a full stomach

Nap/quiet time	12.30–1 p.m.	Start of the single nap, if needed Ideally 1–1½ hours+ in duration Allow to wake naturally, or waken by 2.30–3 p.m. at the latest If this starts to interfere with bedtime then limit to 2.30 p.m. If no nap is required, encourage quiet time instead around the timeframe the nap should/would happen – reading or listening to audiobooks, no television
Drink and snack Leisure		Provide drink and healthy snack on waking up Ensure high-level activity in the afternoon
Dinner	5–5.30 p.m.	Provide dinner with meat protein and carbohydrate
Fixed feed	5.45–6.15 p.m.	Provide bedtime drink/snack, if applicable Do this away from the bedroom with the lights on, so it has nothing to do with sleep
Bedtime routine	6.20–30 p.m.	Start of bath and/or bedtime routine in the bedroom where your child will sleep
Into bed	6.50 p.m.	Have your child climb into bed Use the stay-and-support approach as required
Aim to be asleep	7 p.m.	Aim for your child to be asleep for 7 p.m., with no more than a 4–5 hour window of wakefulness between the end of the nap, if your child is still having one, and being in bed asleep If dropping the nap and your child is visibly tired, you may need to bring bedtime forward to 6 p.m. onwards, adjusting everything by one hour or the corresponding amount Initially aim for 7 p.m. but as your child gets better rested and a later bedtime emerges, start to prepare for bedtime 45 minutes before this time

If your child routinely falls asleep later then you can start to adjust bedtime as follows.

	For a natural bedtime of 7.30 p.m.	For a natural bedtime of 8 p.m.
Bedtime routine	6.50 p.m.	7.20 p.m.
Into cot	7.10 p.m.	7.40 p.m.
Aim to be asleep	7.30 p.m.	8 p.m.

Chapter 10

Feeding

Food and sleep are deeply interrelated. From the moment our children are born, focus is high on ensuring they are getting enough to eat in order to gain weight and thrive. Regardless of your chosen feeding practice – breast or bottle – all any parent wants is for their child to be satisfied.

Fear of waking due to hunger is ingrained in parents from early on. Encouragement to 'fill your baby up' so they will sleep longer is common. Yes, your child will of course wake to feed when they are hungry, but they will wake for many other reasons too – if they are not warm enough, if they are uncomfortable, if they want to connect with you, if they have had enough sleep or they are overtired. For newborns, it is fair to say that hunger governs sleep tendency. Due to their small stomach size, they may wake and feed often in a 24-hour period.

This dynamic reduces significantly after the four-month mark, when the character of sleep starts to lock into place, your baby's stomach size increases and the ability to drink more, less often, and to sleep longer is constantly emerging – if allowed.

Drinking a bottle or having a breastfeed directly before bedtime can have an unwanted effect on sleep ability – this is explored at length in Chapter 2. That is not to say that you shouldn't feed to sleep – you must do what feels right for you – but understanding its impact on sleep tendency may help you make an informed decision about the timing of the final feed at bedtime.

Up to six months of age, the final milk feed will very likely be before bedtime, and ideally in tandem with my percentage-of-wakefulness approach (see page 64). But if your baby is six months and over and they are still waking frequently overnight, then moving the final feed earlier can have an unexpected positive impact on sleep. You may also need to work on the overnight period, however, as this initial adjustment just paves the way for better sleep to emerge – it doesn't instantly improve the night-time, but it creates the space for it to improve with continued adjustments, as outlined in Chapter 12.

Many parents are surprised that the final milk feed could be undermining their child's sleep ability, as, again, ensuring your child is well fed before bedtime has long been promoted to get children to sleep longer. It can, in fact, create a barrier to your child's ability to cycle through their natural overnight sleep phases, due to the design of sleep and how the brain processes associations at bedtime, and how that can affect the ability to maintain sleep overnight.

This is not to discount the evidence for how breastmilk and/or sucking helps promote relaxing and sleep qualities; but we need to take the science of sleep into account also.

We will continue to provide a feed close to sleep time for as long as desired by the parent, but creating a greater distance between finishing that feed and actually going to sleep may make a significant difference.

Lucy Says

In a recent poll of parents that made this adjustment alone, 56 per cent reported an improvement in their child's sleep. While that leaves 44 per cent that reported no changes, it is still one single adjustment with the potential to improve sleep tendency in more than half of the children whose parents made it.

Q *But won't my baby be hungry?*

I would never suggest anything that would further undermine your child's sleep. Many families are feeding very close to sleep time and baby is still waking frequently, so it's not hunger that's the problem. As your baby gets older, it is the brain that sleeps, not the stomach. That doesn't mean that hunger doesn't impact sleep – it just doesn't impact it as greatly as you may imagine, especially as your child gets older.

Furthermore, hunger – or not feeling full – should be addressed at meal settings and throughout the day, not just in the last few minutes before sleep. Relying on a solitary milk feed at bedtime to carry the can doesn't seem reasonable, so we must consider intake on a 12–24 hour basis and create a balance between feeding and sleeping so the rhythms of both run alongside and promote each other.

The goal is to ensure your baby is well fed *and* well rested *and* connected, creating a positive cycle that helps all members of the family.

Lucy Says

When we adjust the feed, it is only by about 45 minutes to an hour earlier – that should not make your baby hungrier, but it may help them to sleep longer, as sleep ability will have the chance to emerge together with other necessary adjustments.

Fixed-feed concept

Q *My baby refuses to take much of the feed earlier/only wants the feed when the lights are out/is too distracted otherwise*

When addressing a feeding-to-sleep association because it is creating a barrier to better sleep, I encourage parents to leave the feed behind by 6.15 p.m. with my fixed-feed concept, even if your child doesn't drink much. This is ideally done in the living space, in bright light and in day clothes. The fixed feed is offered between 5.45 p.m. and 6.15 p.m. and then I move on with the bedtime routine. This may mean you need to be brave. You may have to sideline your misgivings about hunger, understanding that the frequency of waking shows they are not routinely hungry within such short periods of time from being fed, but that very possibly they just can't get through their sleep phases. By repositioning the feed, you create a better space and opportunity to stay asleep longer before the next feed – be that overnight or not until morning, based on your child's age – or at least you create the fertile ground for this to grow.

Many parents understand the concept but still bring the end of the bottle up to the bedroom to make sure their child finishes it, and again, while you must always do what feels right for you, this may undermine your efforts. I recommend that you leave it behind.

Recently, I gave a presentation covering all my suggestions. At the end, a mum approached me and said her child routinely woke at 2 a.m. She had done an earlier bedtime, a later bedtime, a longer nap, a shorter nap, but still he woke every night at this time. I asked her if any of my suggestions made sense to her – she replied that she was doing everything that I recommended. So I asked her when did she offer the last bottle. She said just before he goes to sleep. Aha! I replied. Therein lies the answer – or part of it at least.

UNDERSTANDING IS KEY

To successfully uncouple the final feed from sleep you need to understand why you should do so. Drinking from the breast, bottle, sippy cup or water bottle too close to sleep time enables your child to go to sleep with ease but can disable staying asleep without requiring more of the same or routinely waking when you feel they could sleep longer, based on age and stage. What happens at bedtime specifically is what the brain will routinely search for through the night.

Lucy Says

Sometimes, to improve your child's sleep, we need to create what I call 'dramatic distance' between the final feed and sleep time.

Your baby may not take much at the fixed-feed time, but they will initially likely feed again overnight and so can make up any deficit. Very quickly, this can be recalibrated into the daytime intake, and often their willingness to drink more before you begin the bedtime routine improves too, once they realise the fixed feed is the last offer of milk or water before bedtime. It is a case of adjusting their associations.

The same applies for babies who are potentially distracted, fail to stay on task, need the dark and so on. These are just conditioned behaviours that we are modifying. Although I don't suggest turning out the lights, I do encourage a calm and less distracting environment, albeit not in the bedroom, to help them focus. And I also ensure that throughout the day plenty of opportunities to eat and drink are provided, thus giving you the confidence to offer the feed, remove it by 6.15 p.m., regardless of intake, and then commence your formal bedtime routine.

Drip feed by day

Q *My child only drinks little and often through the day*

You may need to try and improve this dynamic, otherwise the cycle of grazing all night is reasonable and to be expected.

Lucy Says

This can be a daunting cycle to reverse, but it can be done in a very short space of time – I do this routinely with families in my practice and will cover here what you can likely anticipate.

Commonly, when a child drip feeds by day, they don't take enough of the bottle or breast when offered. Worried about hunger and intake, parents then routinely offer feeds over the course of a few hours or throughout the day, so all the feeds merge into one another. Generally, parents will report their child taking little and often, not eating much solid food and then drinking in the same capacity or more overnight.

Many families report very little milk intake by day and the lion's share of the milk intake overnight. Many also suggest that their child has a 'hit or miss' attitude for eating food – not always but often.

Let's try to examine all the dynamics. First, we need to establish what your child's current milk intake should be based on age. We then need to reposition the majority of that intake, if not all, when age appropriate, into the day, with fewer or no calories, based on age/what your child may need, at night.

If you're unsure about intake and amounts, discuss it with your GP or health visitor so you are applying an appropriate approach for *your* baby.

The following is a guideline only, although many parents are surprised at how much the amount of milk required reduces over the first year, and many families are experiencing an over-reliance on milk feeds, which interferes with both sleep and appetite.

Age	Milk intake	Number of feeds	Solid food amount
6–7 months	26–32oz 680–840ml	4–6	Introduce breakfast, lunch and dinner as appropriate
7–12 months	16–21oz 420–630ml	3–4	3 solid meals, 1–2 containing meat protein 2–3 healthy snacks
12–18 months	8–14oz 210–400ml	2–3	3 solid meals, 1–2 containing meat protein 2–3 healthy snacks
18m+	5–8oz 150–210ml	1–2	3 solid meals, 1–2 containing meat protein 2–3 healthy snacks

Ideally you would start to observe my age-relevant feeding and sleeping suggestions (see Chapter 9) and provide the milk and the solid food as outlined. This is can be hard to do if the breast or bottle is also used to achieve daytime sleep.

To begin to reverse the cycle, two things usually need to happen:

1. Milk before sleep – at bedtime and then at naptime – needs to be uncoupled

2. The offering of feeds by day, and then overnight, needs to be regulated as appropriate

---

Lucy Says

It can be hard to regulate daytime feeds when nursing or bottle-feeding to sleep by day. This way you are feeding at the feed times suggested, but you are also feeding to induce sleep, which continues the over-reliance on milk by day and by night and also suppresses the appetite for solid food.

Disproportionate feeding cycle

Countless parents who attend my practice are in a disproportionate feeding cycle. They report feeding and sleeping issues. Most of the time the work we do on the sleep helps to reverse the disproportionate milk-feed cycle, providing for correct milk intake by day and by night, as appropriate, and unlocking the appetite for solid food.

When there is an over-reliance on milk, the appetite to eat solid food is compromised. And when milk feeds are offered too frequently, the appetite for main meals is affected, and this further contributes to sleep issues, as your child may not sleep well because, while not necessarily hungry, they do not feel full or satisfied on a high percentage of milk and a low percentage of solid food.

This is tricky territory, as from birth upwards milk is the primary source of nutrition, and then by six months solid food is introduced to complement the milk intake, but with milk – breast or formula – still being the most important nutritional component. However, from nine months on, the roles start to reverse and solid food begins to take over from milk as the main source of nutrition. Ideally, the milk intake will start to reduce – not drastically, but by enough for your baby to get enough to eat *and* drink with all nutritional requirements being met – so that by 12 months on they're having less milk and more solid food in general.

Over-reliance on milk long term – often to make up for missed meals – affects the appetite for solid food and may, in time, affect iron absorption levels, which can increase sleep disruption. Lack of iron is a significant issue in young children anyway, so care must be taken to ensure that iron-rich food is offered routinely.

It is a lot to balance for us parents, but we can do our best to be informed. And we can apply the following positive feeding practices, which will also support positive sleep practices. Most children from six to eight months can tolerate a three- to four-hour milk-feed cycle. This does not mean that you make your baby go hungry by pacing feeds, but, whether your baby is breast or formula fed, they can be expected go longer than before without milk. This would also be complemented with solid-food introduction. If you are feeding to sleep for naps, this is harder to establish, so it is best implemented while making the other adjustments for sleep for your particular issues.

Case study

Harry is seven months old. He is breastfed and has solid food including meat protein in his diet. He is fed to sleep at bedtime, wakes four to six times through the night and is nursed each time he wakes. He is nursed to nap too. His naps can be hard to achieve and they range from 30–90 minutes long. He usually has three naps but can miss the final nap, meaning that his naps can be finished by 2 p.m. or 4.30–5 p.m. He is normally asleep by 7.20 p.m. having been nursed and transferred to his cot already asleep.

His day currently looks like this:

- Wake 6–7 a.m. – not interested in feeding, offered breast, then breakfast
- Nap attempt 8–8.30 a.m. – nursed then transferred to cot, may sleep for 30–75 minutes
- Up and active – offered breast and snack

- Offered lunch 11.30 a.m.
- Nap attempt 12–2 p.m., depending – nursed then transferred to cot asleep, may wake after 30–90 minutes, may be resettled if he wakes early
- Offered breast and snack
- Third nap in buggy – 40–60 minutes, may miss this three out of seven days
- Dinner 5.30 p.m. – main meal
- Begin bedtime 6.45 p.m. – nursed to sleep by 7.20 p.m., sometimes earlier if nap 3 is missed
- Wakes frequently, 4–6 times (sometimes more) – nursed back to sleep, bed-shares, can be alert around 5 a.m.
- Wake to start day 6–7 a.m. – and repeat

Parent goals:

- Go to sleep without nursing in cot in own room
- Dad can also do bedtime
- Sleep through the night – maybe with one feed
- Nap in cot without nursing or being difficult
- Be happy, content and confident to go to sleep
- Eat better with more structured feeds (Mum wants to stop breastfeeding as she feels this is the problem)

HOW I APPROACH THIS

Harry is currently parent- and breast-orientated in the overall context of his sleep. This makes it challenging for him to sleep through his natural sleep phases without more parental input – nursing and bed-sharing.

There are also timekeeping issues, with naps attempted when he is already overtired, resulting in naps that are short and varied in duration. This means he is under-rested by day – he also often misses a necessary third nap, resulting in a long wake period before bedtime that further exacerbates the issues.

Additionally, there is a likely over-reliance on milk, with frequent day- and night-time feeds and feeds that assists both day- and night-time sleep, explaining why he is not showing interest in solid food. Mum is viewing the breastfeeding as the issue, but it isn't. Hopefully by addressing the actual issues appropriately – uncoupling feeding from sleep at bed and naptime – we can regulate the feeds and decrease the volume of milk to an age-anticipated amount and/or frequency, together with a solids meal plan to suit. This way, Mum will ideally continue to breastfeed and baby can sleep better too. The GP and health nurse have both suggested that no night-time feeds may be appropriate.

To start, we need to establish the age-relevant feeding and sleeping balances for six-to-eight-month-olds. We will address daytime sleep using phase 1 wake-window timing (see pages 101–3) during the day, routinely reinstate nap 3 to observe the nap-gap dynamic for this age (see page 174) and complement this with my bedtime number line (see page 133).

Essentially, we will strengthen the timekeeping element. During the day we plan to start, we will still nurse Harry for naptime, making the bigger changes first at bedtime with the fixed feed, then begin to regulate the night-time feeds, and then the following day we will observe the feeding and sleeping balances, suggestions and naps for the new approach. The feed dynamic will be more easily achieved when nursing and sleep are not enmeshed.

When making the initial changes at bedtime – having been nursed to nap that day and having achieved the third nap and ending it as close to 5 p.m. as possible – we will bring dinner forward to 5 p.m. This will ideally include some meat protein.

Then we will offer the fixed feed downstairs with the lights on, so it has nothing to do with sleep. It is possible that, because Harry is not used to having his last feed at this time, he may not be very interested in it, especially when it is not being associated with sleep. But offer the feed as planned and stop by 6.15 p.m., regardless of intake.

We will proceed with the new formal bedtime routine in the bedroom where Harry sleeps – it will be adequately dark, with no distractions. It will be easier for Harry if Dad does the first two bedtimes. Although neither Harry nor Dad have done this bedtime routine before, it's an opportunity for them to learn the new approach together, and it will make the transition smoother for Harry if Mum stands back. When Mum does do bedtime herself on night 3, it may be best if she wears a newly laundered top.

Following the bedtime routine in Chapter 11, at 6.50 p.m. Dad will turn off lights, music and white noise, if relevant, and place Harry in the cot awake. Then he will use the stay-and-support approach as necessary (see Chapter 3).

Even though Harry will learn the new way at bedtime relatively quickly, he will still wake frequently overnight – if not more frequently – so his parents will also need to begin an overnight plan (see Chapter 12). Remember, all the sleep segments require intervention. Harry is accustomed to feeding back to sleep and sharing the bed with Mum at some stage in the night. We will begin to regulate the night feeds and possibly wean one or both (see 'Night weaning' in Chapter 12).

Next, we will begin to implement the daytime layout for feeding and sleep, starting the morning after the first night. We will now provide milk feeds on a three-to-four-hour basis or when Harry signals that he is hungry. We will start to spend no more than 30–40 minutes per feed or meal – less if he indicates that he is full – and provide the next meal at the next suggested feed time as outlined.

For example, he wakes at 6–7 a.m. and is offered his first milk feed within 30 minutes and breakfast in the next 30 minutes. Based on this, the next milk feeds are offered at 10–11 a.m. and 2–3 p.m. and then the fixed feed at bedtime. The fixed feed doesn't observe the four-hour guide – it is often less to ensure the dramatic distance between the activities of feeding and sleeping.

For this age range, I would typically provide milk first and then solid food at breakfast and lunch. If, in time, by drinking milk first the solid food is refused, we might reverse the order or split the shift half and half. As mentioned above, whenever possible, spend no more than 30–40 minutes on a feed.

Harry's naps will now be timed according to the suggestions outlined in the tables in Chapter 9, using the stay-and-support approach to achieve them (for more about naps and how to master them, see Chapter 14).

Lucy Says

If your baby is routinely drinking more overnight than by day, and you begin to regulate day and night as outlined, occasionally there is a point where your baby is drinking less in a 24-hour period, before the daytime appetite starts to truly emerge – and it will, generally fairly quickly, certainly within three to seven days.

Expected outcomes over the next month:

- As Harry is being appropriately night weaned, he will become more interested in the morning milk feed and eat breakfast soon thereafter.
- Naps are no longer interrelated with nursing and both parents can provide the bedtime routine – place Harry in the cot and he will go to sleep with relative ease.
- Nap 1 will range from 40 minutes to 1½ hours.
- Nap 2 is ideally routinely 1 hour+.
- Nap 3 is still achieved on some days but this can be hard and it's probably ready to be retired. To that end, naps will need to be moved into position – see page 113.
- Harry is nursing every 4 hours and Mum is getting ready to drop the mid-morning feed in preference to having meat protein in the diet.

The milk-feed dynamic from now until 12 months will be a morning feed, an afternoon feed and a feed before bedtime. Over 12 months, potentially, the afternoon feed will be retired. Whenever Mum and Harry feel the need to feed for comfort and connection then they will do so, but they will avoid doing this close to sleep time so they don't undermine their hard work to date. Mum can continue to breastfeed for as long as she actually wants to now that sleep and feeding are no longer interrelated. This demonstrates that it doesn't need to be one or the other – we can continue with a great feeding relationship and improve our sleeping one too.

Chapter 11

Bedtime

Bedtime practices and sleep ability

The bedtime sleep segment is the one with all the power. That may sound dramatic, but it's true. Without a high-level sleep ability at bedtime or if bedtime is addressed too late, when the child is overtired, physically or biologically, many families will continue to struggle with their children's sleep.

To encourage better sleep, you need to try to achieve the highest sleep ability possible at bedtime and do it at the right time for your child's body. This means observing the age-appropriate timings for your child's age range, the nap-gap dynamic and the bedtime number line and ensuring that, if required, you transition from any of the associations at bedtime that do not tend to support more consolidated sleep.

THE BEDTIME NUMBER LINE

- 5 p.m. – dinner
- 5.45–6.15 p.m. – fixed feed
- 6.30 p.m. – bedtime routine
- 6.50 p.m. – into cot/bed

Many parents report that their issues are *not* with bedtime – bedtime is an easy affair.

Lucy Says

I hear all the time, 'Bedtime is not my problem, keeping them asleep is ...'

However, a high percentage of the time, bedtime actually is the problem – it is just not obvious to you. The challenges that you experience overnight, early morning and by day do indicate that bedtime could be part of the problem.

Routine bedtime practices that could undermine your child's overall sleep ability:

- The gap of wake time between last nap and sleep time exceeds the recommended dynamic –even if this is not by much in the overall scheme, it can be the key reason behind continued sleep struggles.
- The day layout is imbalanced/not age relevant and/or the final naps are weaker in the run up to bedtime, leading to biological overtiredness come bedtime, even if it is well timed on paper.
- The daytime sleep has been dropped too soon for your child's age range.
- There is a partial or complete parental orientation at bedtime that is impairing the ability to go asleep with ease and/or stay asleep more and nap better by day.

INCOMPLETE SLEEP ABILITY

This is generally represented by something innocuous that you do before your child goes to sleep. Commonly, the final feed is too close to sleep time. It may be separate, in another room even, but the time between finishing the bottle or breastfeed and being asleep is too short. So if there is less than 45 minutes between the end of feed and sleep, and you are struggling with some element of your child's sleep – be it night-time activity, early waking, nap resistance or short nap durations – this may be the cause.

Any item – a bottle, breast or cup or water bottle – that your child even momentarily sucks on too close to sleep time is an undermining influence on other sleep segments.

Or it could be touching, patting, re-tucking the blanket or a kiss on the forehead, just as they go to sleep, that is affecting their sleep ability.

Q *My child has a bottle at bedtime. He goes into the cot awake but there is probably only 30 minutes between finishing the bottle and being asleep. We continue to have night-time and nap issues – do you really feel this is the problem?*

It is potentially all or part of the problem, so to be sure, repositioning the final feed can help us to establish what is causing what. In my experience, this dynamic does contribute to a lot of sleep problems. It is not a magic bullet, though – routinely, children who don't sleep well for whatever reason are overtired. If the sleep is commonly disturbed, despite well-timed naps and bedtime, then your child is in an overtired cycle and will continue, each day and night, to repeat the cycle until we can diminish it and replace it with better sleep.

Q *We feed our baby to sleep but she sleeps all night thereafter. Do I have a problem?*

No, not to me, and not unless you feel it is one for your family. I am always telling parents, whatever you are doing, however it looks, if it works for you, in whatever format, then continue as you are – provided it feels right and meaningful to you and your child.

As a 'sleep troubleshooter', I focus on the cause when parents have defined the issue, and we take it from there. Many children are helped to sleep in some way at bedtime and still maintain their night-time sleep and nap well by day. Even in this instance, parents may seek support to encourage a higher sleep ability, as they may themselves find rocking difficult as baby gets bigger, they may want to stop breastfeeding or they may be expecting another baby and are keen to encourage a different way of helping their child sleep. So, whatever the motivation to change, my suggestions can help you engage at bedtime in a different way, one that supports high levels of sleep ability and consolidated and healthy sleep practices.

Take what feels right for you and continue to assess the impact on your family unit.

Common bedtime tendencies

Q *I am totally overwhelmed and find even thinking about getting started really difficult. Do I start with naps or bedtime?*

I always, without exception, start at bedtime. To ensure that the bedtime sleep segment is ideally aligned for positive sleep practices, the following are generally required.

Your child will ideally have a bedtime routine, be placed in their cot or bed *awake* and relatively alert and *not* require a parent to stay as they drift off. In the ideal sleep world, it would take 10–40 minutes for them to go off to sleep, and they would not require *any* input from you. This describes the very highest level of sleep ability and working towards that will help you to achieve better sleep overall.

It doesn't have to look exactly like this, as there are many achievable levels, but this is best practice and what we are aiming for, so we can be certain that the sleep ability is high enough to support more consolidated, less interrupted overnight sleep for your child and family.

Lucy Says

Falling asleep quite quickly – under 10 minutes – and not maintaining night-time sleep or napping well by day often indicates being too tired at bedtime, and that something probably helped them get there. A feed or just some low-level parental input can be enough to dilute your efforts.

Whenever we start to make changes it can feel overwhelming and challenging, and sticking with what you already do can feel easier, even if it doesn't actually work. It does take a leap of faith, a high level of commitment and time. You will feel under pressure and emotionally and physically drained and this is where your loving self-care is needed – support yourself, draft in help and share the load as much as you can.

Improving children's sleep is one of the hardest personal improvement cycles, as you come to this already tired and emotional and probably nervous too. Take it in small chunks of time. Be kind to yourself. Keep a sleep journal and day by day, week by week, you will be able to see as well as feel the improvements that are happening. But it does take time.

Q *Oh my god! Every bedtime is different in our house. Some bedtimes are easy – other nights we are up in her bedroom for hours.*

Bedtime can present in a number of ways, and in different ways on different days, and you can spend a lot of time trying to analyse *why?*

These are the common bedtime tendencies:

- It can be easy, looks like no input is needed, parent can leave the room
- It can be easy, requires low input, parent stays: may rub, stroke etc. or just be present; may even have moved away from cot or bed
- It is easy initially but you have to keep returning to the room, doing a 'dance' of coming and going
- You child needs you to be present – you either do something or just be there, can be easy or take hours
- Your child is fed/rocked/walked/rolled in buggy/lain down with to sleep and transfers easily to the cot/bed already asleep
- Your child is fed/rocked/walked/rolled in buggy/lain down with to sleep and takes several attempts to transfer to cot asleep – takes anywhere from 45 minutes to two hours

- You end up bringing them into your bed each bedtime – they start their night sleep in your bed or join you in your bed later in the night
- They resist bedtime – can involve lots of upset and takes anywhere from one to three hours, often parents abort mission and retry, staying, leaving, returning and ultimately staying
- Older children resist bedtime by stalling, looking for extras – require a parent to lie in bed with them

There are many other ways that bedtime can look, but hopefully at least one of these points will resonate with you. More importantly, let's look at how we can address these struggles.

Q I really want to break a feeding-to-sleep association at bedtime

When you know it is a possible problem, then you can start making changes towards greater sleep ability. I outline my own ways of helping to separate the final feed, establish the bedtime and make overall improvements – but what you do at bedtime to help your baby to sleep nearly always must be adjusted if we intend to move forward. Hopefully the information here will show how the way your baby currently goes to sleep at bedtime may need to be addressed if we are to reach your goals.

Getting your child on the correct timing structure for their age range, coupled with the introduction of the bedtime routine with the feed repositioned at the start of the bedtime process rather than at the end, is key. Even if they don't take much at this feed, the important thing is uncoupling the feed from sleep, be it a breast- or a bottle-feed. Utilise the fixed-feed concept (see page 123) and replace what you have been doing to get them to sleep with the stay-and-support method. Continue with the plan overnight and beyond to help address the tendencies that you would like to change.

Q *I am so worried about crying ...*

Crying and sleep have *nothing* to do with each other – your child does not *need* to cry at bedtime or naptime or overnight, but they often do with the introduction of a new skill. Overtiredness can result in your child resisting sleep and having a meltdown around sleep time, and, of course, if you are planning to change how you address any element of your child's sleep, then there may by crying as they process the change.

Learn to understand your child's crying and the terminology around crying and sleep, and if at any time as you make changes it does not instinctively feel right for you, then stop, review and seek out alternative strategies that may sit better with you – you could do this under the supervision of a sleep practitioner so that the recommendations are tailored for your unique family unit.

Just mentioning improving sleep can have strong negative connotations. Parents often refer to 'sleep training', 'cry it out' or 'controlled crying' as possible interventions that improve sleep – and they can do, but these approaches mean you leave your child *alone* following a bedtime routine to process the change and possibly cry, without returning or returning on a timed basis.

These cry-intense methods mean that your child may learn to 'self-soothe', and as a result may sleep better. These approaches can be effective because they are intense and there is very little danger of partial or incomplete sleep abilities because the parent is entirely removed from the context of their child's sleep.

For some, this will work very well. For others, it's not a technique they could imagine using. For others, when they have tried it their child was so upset they made themselves sick or just cried for hours.

Having to address sleep issues is not ideal, and in a perfect world there would not be sleep associations that deplete sleep ability and ultimately require intervention, and our babies would never have to learn or undergo any exercise to improve their sleep. But they often do, and when this is the case, I feel a sensitive, parent-attended approach is more desirable for both parent and baby. So when it is age appropriate to make changes and begin a process, it is done with reduced upset and distress for the child and parent involved.

That is not to say there is no crying – there very likely will be as they process the changes that you make – but they will be supported by you, the parent, and accompanied on their sleep journey, and the foundation for better sleep is put in place before any technique or method is applied.

I cannot tell you that your child won't cry but I can tell you to be available at every step of the way so whatever they experience is with your involvement, which can be gradually reduced over time.

The stay-and-support method is a modified 'gradual retreat', meaning you stay with your child and support them with physical, verbal and emotional encouragement. If your child cries with you beside them, then picking them up to calm them is all provided for. This is not the same as crying it out.

It *is* crying, though, but that is to be expected – it is your child's primary mode of communication, and they will tell you that they are confused, angry, frustrated and annoyed with the new approach. They will protest that the old way suited them better and they will beg you to reinstate the familiar props you had been using – even if that still makes them upset. You are making a *new* familiar by encouraging a slightly different way to achieve sleep, and to do this they will need your support. Change is always hard, but we can adapt – that is the beauty of human nature.

The level of crying, just like sleep itself, has many factors: your child's age, their stage, their temperament, how long the issues have been going on, what you may have tried before, the time you have done this at, whether your bedtime routine was long enough, which parent is trying to make the changes and how emotionally regulated that parent is themselves.

Whatever crying there is, it is always best done with your presence – even when that feels like a distraction. Accompanied crying is preferable, and no crying would be desirable but not realistic, and we do need to manage expectations.

To put crying into context: provided you can say that your child is old enough for change, is clean, dry, warm, loved and not overtired, then their crying is a response to change. Yes, they may have temporarily elevated stress levels, yes, it is not ideal to see them so distressed, but with your presence and support you can lower the stress level and help them to transition from their previous associations towards new ones that will encourage a higher level of sleep ability that will allow them to become optimally rested.

My hope is that crying will be short-lived as your child learns. On night 1, provided it is timed precisely, the process typically takes an hour or so – sometimes longer, sometimes shorter. Bedtime that first night is usually very challenging, but it's also the first improvement area, in that the crying commonly diminishes very quickly over the course of a few days.

As I prefer to avoid crying when possible, it is important that you do not begin using the stay-and-support method until your child is at least six months old. Then it is easier for your child to process the changes and does not result in unnecessary crying that does not diminish and, in turn, does not help to improve your child's sleep.

Lucy Says

It is common for the overall nature of your child's sleep to get worse before it gets better, but provided you are making the key changes and age-relevant choices, everything will start to improve in due course.

Q Is it possible that crying will emotionally damage my child?

There is no evidence to support this, although anecdotally you will hear that crying or sleep training will damage your child psychologically. Many long-term studies have dispelled any concerns, but I suggest that you rely on your gut instinct and that the decisions you make feel appropriate for *you* and *your* family.

Elevated stress levels *do* happen with crying. They are also associated with ongoing sleep deprivation. The anticipated crying is short term as part of an accompanied learning exercise. Sleep deprivation, though, can go unresolved indefinitely if changes are not supported and can affect many aspects of your child's emotional and physical development.

Lucy Says

Not every sleep issue requires a sleep-learning or training approach. Many sleep challenges can be resolved with the age-relevant feeding and sleeping balances and introducing sleep hygiene such as bedtime routines and sleep-friendly environments, all described in this book. However, many of you may also need to change the associations that affect your child's sleep ability and the stay-and-support method will help you make that transition.

It is an emotionally appropriate approach, offering an alternative. So instead of making changes and then leaving it up to your baby to figure it out with you outside of the room (as with cry it out or controlled crying), I promote parental presence and assistance to gently bridge the gap from where you are to where you want to be.

Q *Our two-and-a-half-year-old has recently started having lots of issues at bedtime. She refuses to go to bed. She insists she is not tired and she stalls by looking for water, saying she is hungry and that she needs the bathroom. We are driven demented by this – she and we are up and down the stairs all night, and there is no point in even starting to watch anything before it's time for us to go to bed.*

Limit setting and great timing are the basis of an older child's sleep practices. Things can be trickier as your child becomes more mobile and verbal. It is not unusual for great sleep habits to fly straight out the window when they get a bit older and this, sometimes with the premature introduction of the big bed, can make bedtime a disaster in any household.

If your child is two and a half or younger, then I would strongly encourage the reintroduction of the cot. The challenge under two and a half, and sometimes even when they are a bit older, is that they just won't stay in the bed without a parent anchoring them, and if you try to move through the stages to sleep, they just keep following you out. A better time to make the adjustment to the big bed is closer to three years, and even at that, ideally your child is toilet-trained – this demonstrates the developmental ability to follow instructions, understand and wait – and day sleep has been retired, which usually happens somewhere around age three. If you don't have a nap to worry about, bedtime can be easier and the transition to a big bed smoother.

To establish an older child's bedtime:

- Follow age-relevant timing, as early as is outlined, until going asleep at bedtime is easier and maintaining night-time sleep is better too.
- Reintroduce a nap if visibly tired – in the car or on the couch and over by 2.30 p.m. Don't be afraid to do this, as you're draining the overtired tank.
- The bedtime routine happens in the bedroom – it does not happen in the bed.
- Create a bedtime zone, a visual space in which to do your bedtime routine.
- Have a beginning, middle and end – use a light on a timer to indicate the end of the process.
- Be consistent around requests for drinks – encourage your child to put their cup or bottle into the sink or dishwasher and say goodnight to it. This can help them understand and be part of the concept that drinks are finished for the day, which helps with the separation of drinking from bedtime and overnight.
- Escort them to the bathroom with little fanfare and have little interaction once the lights go out.
- Use the stay-and-support approach for children in a bed and follow the stages, understanding that when your child is older it can take longer and be slightly harder to work through the issues. (For a full plan on older children refer to *The Baby Sleep Solution*, Chapter 6.)

Q What is the best way to bring forward bedtime if you have routinely had a later one?

I bring forward bedtime in one go – I don't do it gradually. On the day that you plan to start, make sure you have your regular wake time – between 6 and 7.30 a.m., no later – and run the day in accordance with your age-appropriate feeding and sleeping balance. If you are planning to create sleep ability that day, cut the naps to the times suggested, using your usual strategies for sleep (you'll make the bigger required changes at bedtime), and provide dinner as outlined, then the final feed and the bedtime routine you have prepared for. *Then* you will use the stay-and-support approach as required to help your child transition.

Some practitioners bring forward bedtime slowly, but once your child is over four months and you control the day as outlined, they are biologically programmed to achieve an earlier bedtime, so I hijack that need with immediate effect.

Q My 16-month-old who won't settle without one of us sitting next to his cot and it's taking up to 90 minutes for him to fall asleep. The nap-gap ratio is right and he shows signs of being tired but he won't settle to sleep on his own.

The nap-gap dynamic may be correctly aligned, but is your child on the right daytime schedule for his age? At 16 months, taking a long time to achieve bedtime could mean you are on one nap a day too soon. As described in Chapter 14, there are certain tendencies that indicate your child is ready for one nap. If this applies, then that is fine but I would recommend looking into that.

Common factors that cause sleep resistance are:

- Overtiredness
- Lack of preparation (bedtime routine)
- Batteries recharged with final feed or screen time
- Overstimulated by the parent's presence

So ensure your child is on the right timings by day and that you precisely follow the fixed-feed concept, nap-gap dynamic and bedtime number line. Have no screen time from an hour beforehand and no feeding close to sleep or becoming too relaxed on their last bottle/breastfeed; have a calm bedtime routine, without siblings and with just one parent.

Initially, place your child in his cot at 6.50 p.m. and use stay-and-support only to achieve sleep. Quickly move through the stages to sleep outlined in Chapter 3 so that you are addressing all possible factors – the key one here is possibly being overstimulated. Ultimately, leaving your child on their own to go to sleep will stop you from acting as an inadvertent barrier to sleep. He may find this challenging but you will continue to support him as you gradually move away through the process.

Lucy Says

It is also possible that his natural bedtime is later. If after two weeks of precisely applying the timings a time keeps appearing that he is routinely asleep by – for example, every night by 8.20 p.m. – then adjust the start of bedtime to 40–50 minutes before this time and see if that adjustment, together with not being as present as before, can help shrink the time it takes for him to go asleep. If starting bedtime later forces everything later, then reverse and stick with what you know.

A typical length of time to fall asleep at bedtime and naptime is 10–40 minutes. Of course, every child is different – some children routinely take an hour, and that is their way. You just need to help them spend that hour managing sleep themselves rather than with you stuck in the room.

Q *I have tried to make the changes but my baby daughter is just so upset. How much crying is too much?*

Adjusting to the changes can be really hard for some babies, and trying to make changes before your baby is old enough makes it almost impossible. Trying to use a sleep strategy before six months can be pointless, which is why I like to think of sleep in two parts – before six months and after.

To make it easier for everyone, ensuring your child is over six months before starting the plan is important. Getting enough sleep by day is also key, so that the night you begin your child is not overtired and their brain is open to learning. The non-breastfeeding parent generally needs to start this process, as having the breastfeeding mum at hand will not be helpful in encouraging a different way to achieve sleep. The main causes of extreme crying are overtiredness and lack of preparation. So ensure that you are addressing both correctly.

Make the bedtime routine at least 20 minutes long – more if you find it is hard to engage with her – in the bedroom where your child will sleep. Before you start this, you will have provided the final feed in the living space and ensured that she didn't get too relaxed during it, as this can often cause a recharge of the batteries, prolonging sleep onset and causing lots of crying.

Some children are very averse to change, so as you accompany them on the journey, you may have to assess it if is too challenging for now and revisit it at a later stage. Understanding the source of the crying helps and being available to support her at all times is key. As with any of my recommendations, if it doesn't feel instinctively right, then search for alternatives that sit better with you.

Crying and sleep have nothing to do with each other. Children do not need to cry to go to sleep – but they may cry if you change what you normally do. This is a protest cry, a cry that overlaps needs and wants – it is their primary mode of communication and their way of processing the change, so the changes must be done with your support, compassion and empathy. The majority of babies can be comforted, and the crying cycle will ebb and flow. Using all my supports – distraction, physical and verbal reassurance and picking up to calm (see pages 26–33) – will help you both master this learning achievement and open the channels for the overnight sleep segment and naps.

Key bedtime adjustments:

- Age-relevant feeding and sleeping balance change
- Nap-gap dynamic for your child's age range
- The bedtime number line
- Stay-and-support approach as required or leave your child to

achieve sleep on their own provided they are calm. If they are not calm, which could happen when you make the changes, use the approach and move through the stages to sleep (as outlined on pages 33–39)

Case study

Twenty-month-old Hannah's parents sought my support to help improve bedtime and overnight in their family. They reported that bedtime started at 7.30 p.m. She would run around for a while, delay on the stairs and play games, together with stalling tactics. Dad did bedtime 80 per cent of the time and would provide a story in a rocking chair. He would then place her in the cot with a hand on her – she could range from being upset to banging her head to being calm. It could take anywhere from 10 minutes to an hour for her to go to sleep. Generally, she would be asleep by 8.30–8.45 p.m.

Once asleep, she might have a dummy resettle at 12.30 a.m. and wake again at 3.30 a.m., very alert. She might be quickly resettled three nights out of seven and take over an hour four nights out of seven. Sometimes this involved walking about with her, giving her water or bringing her into bed. She would wake at 6–6.30 a.m. to start the day. She was in crèche Monday to Friday, with naptimes at 12.15 and of varying duration (from 30 minutes to over two hours). Very often the nap was over by 2.30 p.m., with dinner at 6.15 p.m. and the bedtime routine started at 7.30 p.m. as above.

Mum was expecting another baby, so the main aim now was that bedtime would not be an ordeal. They were also aiming for her to sleep through and to go asleep on her own and not cry for hours as she had been. She was in a cot in her own room but had co-slept until six months – this transition had been made by the parents themselves.

I could see that she was developing typically and there were no red flags there. Her daytime sleep started too early in the crèche and, due to the varied lengths, was often over too early in the day. The bedtime process started too late, when she was overtired, and she was non-compliant – probably due to overtiredness – and parent-dependent so her sleep ability was incomplete at bedtime. Due to both her irregular nap schedule and later onset of sleep, her night waking was unpredictable.

The plan was to continue to observe a wake time between 6–7.30 a.m., no later; create a feeding and sleeping balance for her age range (see Chapter 9); and move the nap, with the crèche's cooperation, to commence routinely at 1 p.m. – this then could finish closer to 3–3.30 p.m.

We brought forward bedtime, and although, as a working family, this put them under pressure, with Mum home by 5.30 p.m. but Dad not home until 6–7 p.m., we still committed to making the changes. We started on a weekend so we would not be under as much pressure. Dad invoked some flexibility in leaving work slightly earlier the following week so that we could give this our all.

She napped from 1 p.m.–3.30 p.m., we brought dinner forward to 5.30 p.m. and all drinks over by 6.15 p.m. We commenced a new bedtime routine in Hannah's bedroom for 6.30 p.m. We created a bedtime zone, had an alarm to signal the start of bedtime and a lamp to signal the end. We gave her lots of choices to stop the stalling tactics, and we indulged in a lovely connected bedtime routine in her bedroom exclusively. We put her into the cot at 6.50 p.m. and used the stay-and-support approach. There was some upset, but Dad supported her, and it took 40 minutes to go to sleep. This meant she was asleep at 7.30 p.m., a whole hour or more sooner than she normally would be. That first night she just had two dummy runs and woke at 6 a.m. Mum and Dad felt positive.

Dad did bedtime nights 1 and 2 and Mum did bedtime nights 3 and 4. This made Mum nervous, as Dad had done the majority of bedtimes to date and routinely Hannah had rejected Mum. But as Hannah became invested in the new approach and was less tired at bedtime due to her later nap and getting more and better sleep overnight, the overtired tank began to drain.

The nap-ending timing continue to vary, but as it did, we collected the data, which demonstrated that she needed four-and-a-half hours' wake time between the end of day sleep and bedtime. When necessary, we started bedtime earlier or later to accommodate this. Mum and

Dad were able to start moving through the stages to sleep into the middle of room on night 7, and by night 13 they were in hallway where she could see and hear them, but at that stage bedtime was an easy exercise for all involved. By night 11 Hannah began to sleep through the night with either one dummy run or none at all.

By night 21 all seemed well, but bedtime regressed. It was possible that she was getting less time for the bedtime routine so we reviewed this and began to ensure that she had positive connected time with Mum or Dad before sleep and that we continue to time bedtime accordingly. I adjusted the bedtime number line to accommodate four-and-a-half hours of wake time, so when the nap ended at 3 p.m., the bedtime routine started at 6.50 p.m. with lights out about 7.10 p.m. and Hannah generally asleep by 7.30 p.m. All was routine and ready for baby number two in October!

Chapter 12

Overnight

Common overnight issues

Overnight issues regularly reported by parents include:

- Frequent night-time waking – sleeping well until 10–11 p.m. and then starting to wake every 40 minutes to two or three hours
- Waking every 40 minutes to two hours from bedtime, rarely ever sleeping for more than two hours at a time
- Waking and staying awake for a long period of time, one to three hours
- Waking really early to start the day – may or may not have woken frequently before being ready to get up at silly o'clock
- Will only return to sleep with milk – breast or bottle – or you may have replaced this with water but the waking continues
- Will only return to sleep in your or the spare bed – may also demand milk or water

Parents, of course, want to know how to stop various tendencies overnight, but as I hope you've seen in the earlier chapters, what happens in the overnight sleep segment is very often governed by the other sleep segments, resulting in symptomatic waking – waking caused by what happens at bedtime and by day and then ingrained into overnight as a result.

Sometimes parents say, 'I know it is only a habit or for comfort', but I feel it is always more than that and that children are entitled to wake for comfort, reassurance, connection and feeds when they are required.

Lucy Says

Whatever happens overnight is a representation of the associations your child may have in relation to their overall sleep. For example, if they feed to sleep – breast or bottle – they may 'need' to feed back to sleep overnight to help them through their night-sleep phases. They may also feed from a legitimate need and look for support from you, as being away from you overnight is a long time.

Sometimes the need to feed back to sleep is historic, as in, it was necessary and just never went away due to associations at bedtime or nap deprivation by day.

The night waking, however, may be because of the overtired tank always being too full. As we've seen throughout this book, being overtired contributes hugely to many of the issues you may observe:

- Frequent dummy re-plugs
- Frequent waking to be settled or fed
- Restless sleep
- Long wake periods
- Early rising

The above, and more besides, all can be attributed to being under-rested from not getting enough sleep and/or having continued disturbed sleep. The frequent dummy re-plugs do not mean you have to stop using a dummy – the more rested you can help your child to become, the less you will need to do. That doesn't mean that you won't have dummy re-plugs here and there, but you can dramatically reduce them once you start to make the changes I propose.

As before, how you achieve and attempt to maintain their sleep forms their associations with what they need or want to get back to sleep overnight.

Lucy Says

There is generally little point in addressing the overnight sleep segment if you have not made the necessary changes at bedtime, both in terms of timing and application. Remember, the bedtime sleep segment controls sleep ability's emergence overnight. Even if you feel you have no issues with bedtime, I strongly encourage you to read Chapter 11 so you are certain the correct parameters are in place to ensure sleep success overnight.

If what you are currently experiencing works for you, even if it is outside of my suggestions, that's fine – remember, there is no right or wrong way. But if you desire change, then there is opportunity. Using this book to help piece your plan together will help in achieving your goals. With my first book, *The Baby Sleep Solution*, many parents reported being too tired or not having enough time to read a whole book. I encourage you to make time to read all of this one. I have tried my best to make it easy for the tired brain, linking the segments and common queries together, but working through everything is part of the solution. Consider taking time to read the whole book as a part of your own self-care, because once sleep starts get better, then I find the whole family unit can operate optimally.

Remember, we are not necessarily looking for sleeping through the night. We are realistic and mindful of expectations sometimes exceeding a baby's capability. Remind yourself of this frequently so you are not reaching for the unattainable, just seeking better than you currently have.

Furthermore, if you make changes to the daytime and bedtime but you do not actively address the night-time activity in an appropriate way, then the reported issues may continue, so action on the overnight segment is very important.

Resolving night waking

🅠 *My son wakes loads overnight. We don't feed him, as we know he doesn't need a feed, and even if we give one, he is not interested – he just keeps waking. We give him the dummy, turn him on his side, rock or cuddle him back to sleep. Most of the time, by 4 a.m. he comes into my bed, and even at that he is still restless.*

If you currently address your overnight without feeding, then your overnight plan is actually quite simple. I will assume that you have made the necessary adjustments at both bedtime and through the day to ensure that you are either enhancing sleep ability at bedtime or maintaining it, as outlined in Chapter 11. This, coupled with the age-relevant feed and sleeping suggestions, means that you have a higher chance of now being able to help your child sleep better overnight.

Once he has gone to sleep at bedtime – whether you needed to use stay-and-support or could leave – any time he wakes between bedtime and 6 a.m. you must resettle him using the stay-and-support approach. If he wakes and it is just a dummy run, put it in his hand, guide it to his mouth and leave. If he is more wakeful, return to his room, position yourself beside the cot or bed and use the stay-and-support approach each and every time.

This may mean he stays awake for longer than normal or that he's upset, as you normally bring him into your bed.

Lucy Says

Whatever you normally do or have done – be it cuddle, pick up, walk about, re-plug, flip, bed-share – you replace with the stay-and-support approach. Each night you apply this, you are working away from their current expectations overnight towards new ones, with an increased sleep ability that then promotes further sleep ability into the daytime and the end of the vicious overtired cycle.

Be very careful that if your child wakes early to start the day you still use the approach precisely, so you do not ingrain early activity (see Chapter 13).

Remember, also, that moving through the stages to sleep while using the stay-and-support method is very important, so refer to Chapter 3 too so you do not remain in the first stage of sleep learning and, in turn, don't make the progress you would like.

For ease, I propose that overnight for the first seven to ten days you stay in the stage 1 position, beside the cot, for all night-time waking. Although you may have started to move away from the cot at bedtime and naptime, more support is generally needed overnight so commit to this initially. You may find that before you start moving away the night waking is already gone or very much diminished. If not, by night 14 try to synchronise the position overnight with how you operate at bedtime and naptime, so less of everything and further away. Be careful that you don't create an expectation to be turned on their side or re-tucked overnight, as this may replace what you have adjusted away from.

Night weaning

Q How do I stop providing feeds overnight?

If it's agreed with your GP or health visitor that your baby no longer needs night-time feeding then, together with making all the other changes to help consolidate the night-time, you can begin a night-weaning exercise.

For night weaning to be effective, your baby needs to not have a biological night-feed requirement and to have a complete sleep ability (or one that you are working on) at bedtime and daytime. Your bedtime needs to be in line with my suggestions, and you will need to ensure the final feed is already entirely separate or you are establishing this with the fixed feed.

If you are starting to make all these changes, then we will work on the overnight at the same time – acknowledging that addressing overnight may take the longest in terms of improvement. The decisions that you make and how you operate overnight during this time frame can really make the difference between the approach working or not.

NIGHT-WEANING SITUATION 1: MULTIPLE OVERNIGHT FEEDS

Your baby feeds on multiple occasions overnight – breast or bottle. They take lots of short feeds or lots of long feeds but there is consensus that this is no longer required. They may feed and be returned to their cot or they may feed and bed-share, but you are also actively looking for them to sleep in their cot all night.

To begin:

- ☑ Regulate the night-time feeds by deciding that on night 1 you will only provide the feed on a four-hour basis.

- ☑ If your child wakes less than four hours from the bedtime feed – note: not sleep time but the final feed, which will likely be 5.45–6.15 p.m. – do not offer a feed.

- ☑ If it is a dummy re-plug, put it into their hand, guide it towards their mouth and leave.

- ☑ If it is more than that (they are more wakeful) then resettle them with the stay-and-support approach – even if you did not need to implement this approach at bedtime you will need to support them in a different way now to replace your original activities.

- ☑ On their first wake at least four hours after the bedtime feed, provide the first night-time feed.

- ☑ If you are bottle-feeding, make the same amount that they normally drink – 150ml or 210ml, for example; if they have been only drinking small amounts on multiple occasions through the night, provide 210ml and they can take what they want when offered on this occasion.

- ☑ If you are breastfeeding, then actively unlatch after the first 10 minutes on one or both sides, depending. If your feed time is longer normally, then cap at 10 minutes; if it is shorter, then work off this time (typically five to eight minutes max anyway) and reduce to two to three minutes by night 3.

☑ Then run the four-hour parameter again – if they wake within four hours of the first night-time feed, resettle them with the stay-and-support approach as needed; if it is just a dummy resettle, put it into their hand, as above, and leave.

☑ On their first wake at least after four hours from the first night-time feed, provide a second night-time feed. Once again, provide the same amount as for the first night feed.

☑ For any waking after the second feed until 6 a.m., resettle using the stay-and-support approach.

☑ Treat any time before 6 a.m. as night-time. If your baby is awake before 6 a.m. then use the stay-and-support approach, even if they really won't return to sleep – we never start the day before 6 a.m.

☑ Beyond 6 a.m., get up and start the day. If your baby has been awake from an earlier time, do an exaggerated wake-up, where you leave the room for a second or two and return with a 'rise and shine'.

☑ If your baby stays asleep, remember to wake them by 7.30 a.m. to regulate the day.

Over the next few nights on both feeds, reduce the *amount* in the bottle or the *time* on the breast by actively unlatching as follows:

- Night 1: 210ml/10 minutes
- Night 2: 120ml/6 minutes
- Night 3: 60ml/3 minutes
- Night 4: no night-time feeds – use stay-and-support for any and all night-time waking

Lucy Says

This is definitely a challenging part of helping to reduce night-time activity. It will require confidence around hunger and patience around upset and a level of distress as your child processes the different way you are handling night-time from now on.

It is really important that, if possible, the breastfeeding mum *does not* attempt the settling without feeding and only appears for the feed. The other parent is highly encouraged to take on the settling job, as ultimately it will be easier for the baby to acclimatise if Mum is not present. Again, you must do what feels right, but it tends to be unhelpful if Mum attempts to do the settling. If Mum must do it, then she would ideally wear a newly laundered top.

Furthermore, if or when your child does not return to sleep on the reduced amount of night feed, then implement the stay-and-support method. On the nights that you begin to reduce the calorie intake overnight, it is usual for your child to stay awake for one to two hours, sometimes more.

Working through this with them predictably and not reintroducing the feed or providing a substitute, such as water, is key. Then you can expect the night-time sleep to start to consolidate – provided you have observed all the other recommendations. Night weaning in isolation may not correct the reported issues, so attention to all the segments and suggestions is essential.

NIGHT-WEANING SITUATION 2: SINGLE FEED BEFORE 12 A.M.

If you are just weaning one night-time feed – breast or bottle – then, depending on when you normally provide the single feed, the plan is adjusted as follows:

☑ If you typically provide the single night feed before 12 a.m., then if your child wakes after 10 p.m. or four hours from bedtime feed then you will offer the single night feed.

☑ If they wake before 10 p.m. or four hours from bedtime feed and it is a dummy run, put it into their hand, guide it to their mouth and leave; if is it more than that, then settle with the stay-and-support method.

☑ On their first wake after 10 p.m. or four hours offer the feed, allow them to drink – they can even fall asleep on this feed – and return them to the cot.

☑ With any waking after this single feed and before 6 a.m., resettle them with the stay-and-support approach.

☑ Treat any time before 6 a.m. as night-time. If your baby is awake before 6 a.m. then use the stay-and-support approach, even if they really won't return to sleep – we never start the day before 6 a.m.

☑ Beyond 6 a.m., get up and start the day. If your baby has been awake from an earlier time, do an exaggerated wake-up, where you leave the room for a second or two and return with a 'rise and shine'.

☑ If your baby stays asleep, remember to wake them by 7.30 a.m. to regulate the day.

Lucy Says

While I typically discourage feeding to sleep, when working on improving sleep, it is OK to allow your baby to fall asleep on this single overnight feed – I am inclined to allow the feed to work for you at this point, as you will be weaning your child from this feed over the next few days anyway.

NIGHT-WEANING SITUATION 3: SINGLE FEED AFTER 12 A.M.

If the single night-time feed is generally offered sometime between 12 a.m. and 6 a.m. then proceed as follows:

☑ Provide a single feed on their first wake any time after 12 a.m. – don't delay this to 3–5 a.m.

☑ If they wake before 12 a.m. and it is a dummy run, put it in their hand, guide it to their mouth and leave; if is it more than that, then settle with the stay-and-support method.

☑ On their first wake after 12 a.m. offer the feed; allow them to drink and return to sleep on the feed.

☑ For any waking after this single feed and before 6 a.m., resettle with the stay-and-support approach.

☑ Treat any time before 6 a.m. as night-time. If your baby is awake before 6 a.m. then use the stay-and-support approach, even if they really won't return to sleep – we never start the day before 6 a.m.

☑ Beyond 6 a.m., get up and start the day. If your baby has been awake from an earlier time, do an exaggerated wake-up, where you leave the room for a second or two and return with a 'rise and shine'.

☑ If your baby stays asleep, remember to wake them by 7.30 a.m. to regulate the day.

FOR BOTH PRE-AND POST-12 A.M. NIGHT-WEANING SITUATIONS:

Over the first four nights, reduce the *amount* in the bottle or the *time* on the breast by actively unlatching as follows:

- Night 1: 210ml/10 minutes
- Night 2: 120ml/6 minutes
- Night 3: 60ml/3 minutes
- Night 4: no night-time feeds – use stay-and-support for any and all night-time waking

Q *My baby will go nuts if we don't give a feed*

Your child may find this element challenging if they have routinely had a bottle or a nursing overnight. Starting the journey towards no night-time feeding can be hard for all involved. By reducing rather than immediately eliminating the amount of the feed over the few nights you can help them to acclimatise and to expect less calories, but even with this adjustment it can be a tough journey.

Ensuring that you have aligned the sleep parameters as suggested will help make this as easy as possible on them, but it will be hard generally either way. As a parent, it is a case of assessing whether night feeding is still appropriate (see below if it is) and what effect the night feeding is having on the overall quality of their sleep – their mood, behaviour and appetite. Often we see a disproportionate feeding cycle, with more milk consumed overnight than by day, and a hit-and-miss dynamic to solid feeding that is being compromised by unnecessary night-time feeds. This is waking the digestive system when it should be resting, filling nappies so they leak or require changing and possibly preventing your child from cycling effectively through their natural sleep phases without lots of parental input. It may also have an effect on their dental hygiene.

Lucy Says

Allowing your child to process this change with your support is necessary. Acknowledging that it will be a difficult adjustment and will probably mean everyone gets less sleep than before is also generally part of the journey. But once addressed correctly, within 7–10 days of no night-time feeds you will likely report much better night-time sleep consolidation, not to mention more appropriate daytime appetites for both milk and solid food, together with enhanced mood and probably better napping too.

Q *Is it OK to give them water instead?*

Generally, I don't suggest providing water instead of the original milk feeds because, although I know they may not be interested in the water, very often the need to drink milk transfers into the need to drink water – even if you use a sippy cup! So I would avoid if possible.

But won't they be thirsty?

Again, we generally don't anticipate night-time thirst, but you as parent must make that call – you probably need to assess from where the drive to drink back to sleep is originating, based on what you have learnt here, and make an informed decision. Again, if you plan to offer water in any capacity, then you may undermine what you are trying to achieve.

Where will I do the feed – we often bring our baby out of the room to make the bottle?

All night-time feeds need to happen in the bedroom and without first taking your baby on a tour to prepare the feed. For the nights while we are discontinuing the feed, be prepared in advance of the waking and offer the feed quickly in the dark in the bedroom where they sleep. Sit in a chair – try not to lie on a bed if breastfeeding – so you can feed and return your child to the cot if this is where you want her to sleep overnight.

If she won't settle should we just give in and provide a feed?

Once we commit to reducing and eliminating the feed, it will undermine the process if you cannot see the night-weaning exercise through. If you allow her to fuss and wait for 40 minutes or an hour and then give her a feed, you are training her to wait and cry and we definitely don't want that.

If you just cannot see it through, then sometimes providing a dream feed before the feed time will help by ruling out that hunger – conditioned or otherwise. This may mean you go back a few paces and provide one or two dream feeds, depending on your journey, and then whenever baby wakes they are only ever resettled, as you have initiated the feeds already. This still means night-time calories and wake-ups, but it can help to diminish the expectation of waking and being fed if you cannot follow through the original process.

A dream or sleepy feed is where you lift your baby from their sleep and initiate a feed – the idea is that you don't allow them to wake and be fed, only ever resettled. This can be a suitable approach when retaining night feeds, as mentioned below, but it is not my go-to approach. I prefer child-led feeding, but I will implement this to overcome not being able to resettle without feeding and worrying about hunger.

- If you provide one dream feed then 11.30 p.m. works well.
- If two feeds are needed then 9.30 p.m. and 1.30 a.m. work well.

Lucy Says

To dream feed, you must initiate the feed, so if they wake before the allocated time, they must be resettled with stay-and-support – then you can lift and feed. They don't need to stay asleep during the feed, they just need to not wake and be fed. This does not completely address night feeds but it is one way to flip expectations and continue to make progress – you can review later what is needed and what is not.

Case study

I recently worked with a family night weaning 10-month-old Archer. He was incredibly upset as the parents tried to night wean and each night, despite their best intentions, they ended up feeding him. This was leading to lots of distress on everyone's part, it was building an expectation to cry and wait and ultimately feed and no progress overnight was being made.

I implemented two dream feeds, initiated by the parents at 9.30 p.m. and 1.30 a.m. Archer still woke and was still really upset, but as Mum and Dad were confident he wasn't hungry and crying for food, they were better equipped to support him. Very quickly, over a few nights, the night-time sleep consolidated and we continued to provide the two dream feeds. The parents didn't feel the feeds were needed, so after two weeks of applying the dream-feed strategy, we began to remove the dream feed at 1.30 a.m. and supporting Archer with the stay-and-support approach. Now there was much less upset, as he already had the skills required to return to sleep without a feed, and this remedied quite quickly. Another week later, we did the same with the dream feed at 9.30 p.m. The end result was consolidated night-time sleep without feeds entirely. We took the scenic route to get there, but with adjustments and a bit more time, understanding and predictability, we were able to achieve the goals together.

🔲 *I still feel that my child needs night-time feeding – how can I consolidate some of the night and continue to feed?*

If, together with your GP or health visitor, you feel night feds are still required, then we can still help your child to sleep between feeds if they currently are waking many times. In this instance, it is important to figure out how many feeds they may need. Assuming your child is at least six months of age, then probably either one or two feeds would be appropriate. I can't tell you what your baby needs unless I am working with you directly, so here you will need to seek support from your own GP or health visitor and, within that, apply the suggestions that resonate with or are applicable to you.

To retain two night feeds, I operate the four-hour window as in Situation 1 (see page 155) – just don't reduce the amount in the bottle or the time on the breast.

To retain one night-time feed, I generally make a decision about what time the feed will be provided –either before or after 12 a.m. as in Situation 2 (see page 157) – again, without the weaning approach

---

Lucy Says

If you allow your baby to wake, be fed and settle in between feeds and the night wakes are still quite high after 10–14 nights, then I convert to one or two dream feeds as outlined in Archer's case study. When this happens, it generally indicates that baby doesn't understand why it is OK to feed sometimes when they wake and not other times. The dream feeds help to overcome this and still night feed appropriately.

Then when you or they are ready, you can always wean by reducing as set out in Chapter 12 and applying the stay-and-support approach.

By allowing a wake-to-feed initially, many children will self-wean – they'll wake later in the night and start to drop the feeds on their own, without your active intervention. If you see this emerging, then I would encourage it.

Very often children under the age of two start to show overnight sleep promise within 14 nights or so – don't worry if you are not seeing improvements this quickly: it is a general observation. But children aged two to four and over often need three weeks or more before you feel like you are breaking ground. Hang in there. Share the load. If not breastfeeding, take the night-time waking in turns and continue to support each other in other ways to proceed through the plan effectively. This may mean allowing one parent to stay in bed in the morning if they have been up a lot overnight. You can decide what works best for you.

I have been making all your changes and the night waking continues – is my child just a poor sleeper?

Some children take longer to improve their night-time tendency, but do your best to be consistent. In my experience, the parents that go off-plan once or twice by providing a feed once weaned or bringing their child back into bed or a bit of both, always take much longer to achieve their goals. The point is to really try your best to be predictable and consistent in the approach. Be very conscious as the nights go by that you are not ingraining the expectation to be helped back to sleep each time they wake; although it is all about support, it is also about creating space and opportunity for your child to stitch their sleep phases together once developmentally appropriate.

At the start of your plan, you should respond quickly and in a large capacity, but as the days go by, it is wise to wait longer, three to seven minutes, before you return to your child so they have the opportunity to return to sleep using their own skill-set and not always with your help. If you originally shared the room, then it is definitely time to move out if you do not plan to be long-term room-sharers. If you are planning to long-term room-share, you may need to assess if you are inadvertently disturbing their sleep while *you* sleep.

It is also important to ensure that your baby is not too hot or too cold – being just right is what is needed, especially in the core part of the night when the temperature drops to its lowest. Make sure the room temperature is moderated to 16–20 degrees and they are dressed warmly enough – in vest and pyjamas as appropriate – and ideally in a sleeping bag to match the season too.

Working through the night-time plan is possibly the hardest part of your sleep journey, as this is where your own defences are low. Share the load as appropriate and know that the investment in this month or so will provide a yield for many years to come.

Chapter 13

Early Rising

Types of early risers

Children who wake early tend to fall into one of five categories:

1. The early learner – this is where you are in the middle of the sleep-learning exercise, making all the changes to improve your child's sleep; as night-time sleep improves, the child wakes early for a few weeks while they learn to cycle through the last and most difficult sleep phase in their overnight sleep segment.

2. The temporary early riser – where your child wakes early out of the blue, having generally slept to 6 a.m. or beyond.

3. The habitual early riser – a child who has become stuck on the last phase.

4. The early starter – a child who is predisposed genetically to waking early.

5. Those who are in an early cycle – bedtime is too early (typically 6–6.30 p.m.) and when they wake at 5 a.m. or so they have had enough sleep to fill their needs.

Waking too soon to start the day can be a vicious cycle and can affect almost any age range. There are certain causes that generally need to be addressed for a child who is a habitual early riser or in an early cycle. With temporary early waking, sometimes the early rising represents something else that may be going on with your child, such as teething or sickness.

Q *My child is awake by 6 a.m. most days – I find it really challenging and would love to stop this early rising!*

Early rising proper is when your child routinely wakes before 6 a.m. to start the day. Many parents describe their child who wakes at 6–6.30 a.m. as an early riser, but typically that is an acceptable wake time for a young child, albeit too early for some of us adults! If this is your child, no intervention is actually required – you just may need to go to bed earlier yourself, in order to be fit for parenting early doors.

Young children are designed to go to bed relatively early and in turn wake early too. The relationship between the bedtime and the wake time is interrelated, but not necessarily in the way that you imagine.

Q *If I move bedtime later will that help?*

Many parents move bedtime later to achieve a later wake time, only to report that their child either wakes at the same time, or indeed wakes even earlier than before! The message here is that the bedtime only controls the wake time to a certain extent.

Lucy Says

Moving bedtime later is more frequently not the answer to achieving a later wake time.

A true early rising dynamic is demonstrated by routinely waking before 6 a.m. to start the day – anything from 4–5 a.m. – and represented by your child having no intention of returning to sleep and enthusiastic to start the day. If this sounds familiar and it has been ongoing for at least six weeks (years for many of you), then you can intervene and make some adjustments to help reverse the early morning waking for many of you.

Q All of a sudden my child has started waking early – originally they woke later but now it's 5 a.m.!

Waking early, out of the blue, having routinely slept later than 6 a.m., when you have had no other changes such as travel or nap transitions, may represent teething, a developmental stage or sickness brewing – this is what I call temporary early waking. No action is required, except to provide a reassuring response, pain medication under the guidance of your GP, and patience. As soon as the phase passes, the early waking will resolve on its own and your previous late sleep will re-emerge, so try not to panic and make unhelpful adjustments. I would be inclined to keep your current timing structure. I would bring bedtime earlier, if anything, and then as soon as the disturbance has passed, your longer night-time sleep tendency will be apparent once more.

Q Do you think that because my husband is an early riser that our child is just the same?

A percentage of children are predisposed to being an early starter by way of genetics. If this is the case, generally one of the parents will be similar. In this instance, it's a case of trying to live with it as best as you can – but always work through the contributory factors, as you never really know until you start to address them whether this is the case for you.

Parents are typically aghast at this dynamic because even if one parent is an early morning person it often won't be as early as your child wants to wake! As your child gets older, there are strategies you can implement to keep them occupied when they are up before everyone else and to prevent them from waking you. I am generally not in favour of these tactics, such as allowing them to play or read, or even get up and begin making breakfast, until you have exhausted all avenues for eliminating the early timings – and you need to be sure that allowing them to play or read will not generate an even earlier wake time, which can start to mean your child doesn't get enough sleep at all.

Reasons for early rising

Understanding why your child may be awake early is the first step in resolving the issue, so let's examine the root causes.

Q *When he wakes early, I often think that he could be hungry – is this a possibility?*

Ruling hunger in or out is often a necessary part of the early rising exploration. Waking early can sometimes be because your child hasn't eaten or had anything to drink for nine or more hours. Providing a milk feed here can sometimes help your child return to sleep if hunger *is* an issue and it is age appropriate – but, especially as your child gets older, it can sometimes ingrain the early waking, as your child becomes conditioned to expect feeding at this early time in the morning. Often parents provide a milk feed or bring the child into their bed and the child still doesn't return to sleep, yet the expectation of an early feed or change in sleep location becomes ingrained, encouraging the early waking, and it can also interfere with your feeding practice for the rest of the day.

Ultimately, you will need to figure out what's causing what: establishing night-time feeding needs can be tricky territory and varies for each child. Once your child is nine months, your task is to ensure that they get enough to eat and drink by day and that their last solid meal is meat protein and carbohydrate based. This can help to keep your child feeling fuller longer and decrease the risk of waking not feeling full.

Lucy Says

However, be cautious about stacking up the calories before bedtime, as this can often undermine, rather than improve, your child's sleep tendencies. As you can see, it is tricky territory!

Using this book, and with your GP or healthcare professional's advice, look at how much milk and solid food is required for your child's age and proceed on that basis. (See Chapter 10 and the recommendations by our expert Caroline O'Connor in Chapter 15.)

If you are operating within a disproportionate feeding cycle – where your child drinks more at night than by day – then Chapter 10 may be particularly helpful, as early rising may be only one part of your current sleep challenges.

DREAM-FEED TRIAL

If you are concerned that providing a feed at 5 a.m. is fuelling the early cycle but are still worried about hunger, trial a dream feed at around 1.30–3 a.m. If your child still wakes at 5 a.m. then it is not necessarily hunger related.

This can be done by setting an alarm (I know – very hard to do!) and then initiating the feed, so you are controlling the expectation and providing the feed on your terms. If you do this and your child starts to sleep later, this could be the answer for you right now. If so, carry on until it starts to affect the first morning feed, which needs to remain established in order for the feeding rhythm by day to stay intact.

When morning-feed refusal starts to happen, reduce the amount in the bottle and/or time on the breast and gradually wean (see Chapter 13) when age appropriate. If your child has started to be able to go longer overnight and is also getting enough by day, then the dream feed can be phased out and your longer sleep phased in.

Q Could the light in the room be encouraging my child to wake early?

Assess the environment, and use darkness to your advantage. Obviously, in the winter months this is not relevant, but certainly from March to October, when the clocks have gone forward, light both at bedtime and early in the morning can dilute your child's sleep efforts.

Around 4–5 a.m. your child will start to commence the final sleep phase. It is the hardest one to complete, as their sleep tank is largely filled, and as a result, something that may seem minor can encourage an early wake-up. Even the smallest sliver of light entering the room from either the hallway or over the top of the blinds can stimulate the waking part of the brain and send a signal that it's time to get up.

Isolate any light sources that may be contributing to this. Blackout blinds are the first solution, best used with a blackout curtain as well. Sometimes this isn't enough either and you need to get creative – perhaps tin foil on the window or another piece of material slung over the curtain pole, and then sealing up any sources of light from the hallway and other areas. Although I do suggest a nightlight in the bedroom, it should only be the dimmest of light sources, and I would take it away altogether if I felt that it was undermining the morning sleep phases.

While you're at it, try to limit other disturbances in the household at this vulnerable time – someone else getting up for work, the dog next door barking, heating clicking on. The chances of these activities signalling it's wake time are pretty high, so be mindful and proactive whenever possible.

I have worked with many families that have to start work earlier than most, and the parents' alarm and their movement can initiate an early waking time. I know it's not realistic, but do try everything that you can to preserve your child's sleep because if you have more than one child, you will know that one up means all up!

Lucy Says

I worked with a radio DJ once who did a morning show and his alarm would most certainly rouse their baby, who was in a light sleep phase. We changed to an alarm that vibrated on his wrist and that helped us somewhat overcome the early waking.

Also, not being warm enough can initiate unwanted early wakes, so plugging all the gaps is significant and ensuring that your child is snug at a time when the temperature will be at its coolest.

Q We are pretty certain that it is not hunger, light or not being warm enough that is waking our daughter, yet she is still awake early – this morning it was 4.45 a.m.!

Often the early wake time is related to what has happened at bedtime: how your child achieved their sleep, what time they went to sleep and the relationship between their final nap and bedtime. This is rather involved but worth working out, as it can make the difference between 5 a.m. and 6 a.m. Let's look at these factors.

Q My child has a bottle at bedtime but stays asleep all night until 4 a.m. onwards – and then is ready to get up and go!

You may need to consider the associations at bedtime to help resolve the early morning issues. Many children have a low sleep ability (see page 19) at bedtime and this dynamic can leave you vulnerable to early waking. When you are completely involved in getting your child to go to sleep at bedtime – transferring your child to the cot or bed already asleep, or staying with them holding hands, nursing or bottle-feeding them until asleep – you are more vulnerable to night-time activity and/ or waking too early (see Chapter 11).

Another typical barrier is an incomplete sleep ability, where the final feed is just too close to sleep time, which enables a sleepy state at bedtime and disables the ability to get through some or all of the night without waking or looking to start the day too soon. As described previously, if your final milk feed is one of the last things you do at bedtime and there is less than 45 minutes between finishing the feed or drink and being asleep, then this is a likely contributory factor to the issue.

To remedy this and the low sleep ability, reposition the last feed or drink before bedtime 45 minutes to an hour before your child will be asleep. This will decrease the risk of early waking and enhance the chance of sleeping to 6 a.m. and maybe even later!

Q *I have established the separation between the feed and sleep time, yet the early waking continues – what can I do?*

All sleep segments affect one another, so we need to work on not only addressing bedtime but also getting enough daytime sleep and making sure that the timing of the daytime sleep and its relationship with bedtime is supporting consolidated, less interrupted sleep and not encouraging early waking.

Early waking is a vicious cycle: your child wakes early, is tired too soon by day because he's awake early, is overtired at bedtime because daytime sleep is over too soon … Using my nap-gap dynamic and bedtime number line will help you to reduce the risks and continue to apply all the suggestions.

Depending on what naps your child needs according to their age (see Chapter 10 on creating the feeding and sleep balance), it can be helpful to observe the following to combat early starts:

- No naps initially before 7.40–8 a.m. following the wake period suitable for your child's age range; after 10–14 days, move nap 1 to 9–9.30 a.m. by five minutes every day (for more on this see Chapter 14).
- Ensure the final naps are over by 5 p.m. (for under eight months) and as close to 3–3.30 p.m. (for eight months to three years) as possible. This can mean delaying nap 2 (eight months and over) to 1.30 p.m. and the single nap (eighteen months and over) to 1 p.m. in order to observe these suggested dynamics.
- Practise smaller wake periods before bedtime (worry less about the ones early in the day). Not observing the nap-gap dynamic (outlined on the next page) before bedtime causes a large share of sleep challenges, including early waking.

THE NAP-GAP DYNAMIC

Age	Hours between nap end and in bed asleep	Suggested nap end time
4–8 months	2–2½	5 p.m.
8–18 months	3–4	3–3.30 p.m.
18–3 years+	4–5	2.30–3 p.m.

Q *What do we do with our child when they wake at 5 a.m. and have no intentions of returning to sleep?*

It's important that as you make the adjustments outlined you treat any time before 6 a.m. as night-time and have a predictable response with the stay-and-support approach. Keeping your child in the dark and in the cot or bed will help them to learn to transition through that last sleep cycle and encourage a later wake time. Unfortunately, even occasional bed-sharing, drinks, TV, phones or iPad use at this time all dig the early-waking hole deeper – ideally you would support your child at this time only with my approach, even if at the start it seems unlikely they will go back to sleep. We don't necessarily expect them to return to sleep, but we want to condition the body to know that 4–5 a.m. is not the right time to get up either.

Lucy Says

By treating this waking with precision, along with the other changes, it will typically take three to four weeks for you to start seeing 6 a.m. or later on your bedside alarm clock, and longer in some instances where the early waking is deeply ingrained. Avoid clocks or other gimmicks designed to help a child sleep later until you have addressed the fundamentals, and even after that I would use them with caution.

LUCY'S CHECKLIST TO COMBAT EARLY RISING

☑ Make sure the room is dark, warm and quiet enough.

☑ Observe the feeding and sleeping balance for your child's age with specific attention to the final nap-gap dynamic above.

☑ Ensure the final feed is at least 45 minutes to an hour before bedtime, offered downstairs with nothing to do with sleep – this is *very* important!.

☑ Continue with your formal bedtime routine.

☑ Use the stay-and-support approach at bedtime if your child requires it because of any changes you have made.

☑ Continue to work through the stages to sleep as outlined in Chapter 3.

☑ Use the same approach early in the morning, avoiding starting the day before 6 a.m., leaving the room, providing drinks or offering your phone.

Stay in Stage 1 (see page 34), beside the cot or bed, overnight for at least 10–14 nights, then start to move positions every three days thereafter as set out in Chapter 3. This may mean you are in a different position for bedtime versus overnight and this is correct. More support is required overnight/early in the morning and this is the part that takes the longest to resolve.

Decide after two weeks if your child would respond better if you didn't enter the room or if you limited the interaction by going in, reassuring and leaving again. Judge this one for yourself. It is easier done if your child is in a cot – in a bed, they are mobile themselves and your presence can help to anchor them.

Understand that you need to be 100 per cent predictable, knowing that one occasion of caving and bringing them into your bed will set you back to the start. Although it is super-hard to stay on track, share the load if possible and focus on the end result.

Q *My day starts too early, then naps are too early, resulting in an early bedtime (asleep by 6–6.30 p.m.), meaning we are in the early cycle you mention – and of course by 5 a.m. they have slept enough.*

Once we begin to address early waking in general then we need to make certain adjustments to stop re-enforcing the cycle:

- From six to eight months: days 1–10/14 avoid naps before 7.45–8 a.m. Once achieving nap 1 relatively easily, then move it forward by five minutes every day, despite your child seeming super-tired from still being awake early. Your goal for nap 1 is at least 9 a.m., and the quicker you achieve this, the better, reducing further the risk factors for early waking. But this can only be done as you improve the night-time, not in isolation.

- From 15 months on: if on a single nap, then initially delay the single nap to 11.30 a.m. with lunch beforehand, then move by 15 minutes every two days until you get to 1 p.m.

- If on one nap a day but unable to cope and seemingly tired before 10–10.30 a.m., then provide a 20–30 minute filler nap in the car or buggy. Wake them and provide the main nap three hours later – commencing the process two hours and 40 minutes after the filler nap has ended. (If you do a filler nap and, as a result, cannot get them to sleep again, you will need to get them to power through the mid-morning by delaying and distracting and adjusting the nap later as above.)

Q *If I delay the naps as you suggest, my child is really tired and they have also been awake for longer than you propose they should be*

Don't worry for the first two weeks of the plan about the gap between waking and the first/single nap being too long – just delay and distract your child as best as possible. This long wake period won't really cause any problems, except that your child will find it a bit hard to wait. It is the gap before bedtime that causes the issues, so that is the one we really need to concentrate on. Every time you allow your child an early nap, the gap is then either too long or you need to provide an early bedtime and therefore end up with early waking for the following day, and we are trying to undo that cycle.

Q How long is this really going to take?

Early waking may take four to six weeks and over to resolve, and you may find that you make all the changes but just don't see a yield. It routinely takes until night 21 and beyond to start to see a change, and even at that it may only be a glimmer. Stick with everything for at least six to eight weeks before deciding that perhaps your child is an early starter by design, which can unfortunately be the case. Don't worry – when they are teenagers, you will take great pleasure in hauling them out of their pit before they are ready, so justice will be served!

In this instance, once you have exhausted all other avenues, I would consider slowly pushing bedtime later, but with caution. Some children can only do 10–10½ hours (and this can be enough for them) and it might be easier for the family if that was 8–6 a.m. rather than 7–5 a.m. However, some children can only achieve their sleep quota on the early timings, and if you move things out at bedtime, the wake time may not change or may get even earlier, creating greater sleep loss and leaving you more vulnerable to an overtired cycle, so judge this adjustment with care.

Ideally, push out bedtime by 15 minutes every three days, in the hope that the extra time gets fixed to the wake time in the morning. If you feel this starts to degrade everything else, then go back to what you know works for now, and focus on all the things that you can achieve early in the morning with your lark ...

Case study

Steve and Laura came to me with their daughter Kate, aged two, to address her long-standing early rising issues.

Kate would wake every morning between 4 and 5 a.m. She would be returned to her bed but kept coming out. Her parents did everything in the morning to keep her resting until 6.30 a.m., but she never went back to sleep.

Her daytime sleep was at about 11.30 a.m. for one to two hours. Bedtime started at 6.50 p.m. and included stories on a rocking chair with milk in a sippy cup. At the end of this she would climb into bed, and they would turn on some music and leave the room. Kate would routinely sleep until 4 a.m. and thereafter would be awake, unable to get back to sleep.

Kate had night-time waking on and off, but the early rising was now the most common dynamic. She had a dummy and a teddy and was in crèche Monday to Friday.

I assessed their case and determined that Kate was developing typically, with no red flags. Immediately, I also saw some timing issues: due to waking early, the nap was too early in the day – the ideal nap is one to two hours long from 1 p.m. onwards. Any earlier means the nap-gap dynamic is too long and the exposure to waking early is valid.

It was possible that getting to 1 p.m. would be too challenging so, with the cooperation of the crèche, we provided a filler nap at 10 a.m. of 20 minutes to get her through the morning, with a main nap offered about 1.30 p.m. If she was coping, we delayed the nap to initially 12 noon and then nudged it later by 15 minutes every day until the nap was at 1 p.m. Lunch was always before the nap and we allowed her to wake naturally, with a cut-off of 3–3.30 p.m.

I also recommended bringing forward the bedtime routine and working off a four-hour wake period until her natural bedtime emerged.

Furthermore, I determined that the rocking chair and milk were putting her into a sleepy state, promoting incomplete sleep ability, although this was not obvious – to her parents she seemed independent at bedtime, as they could leave the room and she would be asleep by 7.15–7.30 p.m.

To address the dependency issues, I changed the order of the bedtime routine, as well as making it earlier and with a shorter wake time before sleep. I told the parents to leave as they normally did provided she was calm.

After the bedtime routine, which was earlier and without the relaxing drink or rocking on the chair, Kate was unable to get to sleep herself and started to get out of bed – this was a clear signal that the dependency existed. So her parents began to use the stay-and-support approach at bedtime. This felt like a regression, as they previously didn't need to stay, but that was only because the milk and rocking were doing all the hard work – enabling bedtime but disabling overnight. So it was actually progress, although it was not obvious as they started.

I did consider her to be too young to be in a bed, but her parents decided to proceed on that basis, understanding that keeping her in the bed without props could be challenging once they were no longer in the first stage of the plan – however, we could review that.

On the first few nights, it took her longer to go to sleep but the input required reduced – now she really was self-settling. By night 4 she had slept to 6.20 a.m. once and we continued to see this emerge – not every day but on and off. Mum and Dad continue to treat any waking before 6 a.m. as night-time and returned her to bed and stayed beside it, using the stay-and-support approach.

The journey was not without challenges, as she found it difficult to stay in bed now that she was no longer anchored by a parent or drink. It took a lot of work but the ultimate goal to enable her to sleep later began to emerge with greater regularity. Some nights she still woke too early, but a consistent response together with all the other adjustments meant that 6 a.m. and later was achieved more often than not.

Chapter 14

Naps

Nap factors

Although I have divided all the sleep challenges into segments in this book, understanding that each sleep segment influences the other is key. Time and again I am asked about specific issues, but each sleep challenge that you experience is part of a bigger picture, and what you report as the problem may only be a symptom – we need to reveal the true cause. Also, some of the reported issues are age based and not a problem per se, although difficult to live through, all the same.

So although you may struggle with napping, the ability to nap *well* is governed by the following factors:

- Your child's age
- The time at which you address bedtime
- When you address the naps
- The length of your naptime routine
- The level of sleep ability your child actually has, both at bedtime and for naps
- What happens overnight
- Where they nap

- When they eat/drink
- Level of stimulation
- How you respond to them before, during and after the nap

Knowing this can stop parents feeling they've tried everything and nothing seems to work. Often it doesn't 'work' because the core contributory factors are not developmentally appropriate or have not been adequately addressed – essentially 'locking out' your child's daytime sleep ability and leaving you frustrated and tired with a plan that doesn't offer a yield.

Lucy Says

The nap-sleep segment is hard to master – it can rarely be achieved without first mastering the bedtime and overnight segments, and it has its own characteristics too. Also, as with everything, it starts off immature and slowly develops as your baby grows so that nap ability changes as your baby does.

Foundations up to six months

Q *My 10-week-old finds it really hard to nap. He totally resists sleep, will only nap on me and if I put him in the cot he will wake up after 10 minutes.*

This is very typical – as outlined in Chapter 5, your child's sleep is immature. Thus they may find it challenging to achieve and maintain their sleep and will look for lots of parental support and only sleep for short bursts at a time in these early months.

It is very typical that a baby fights the nap, needs contact for the nap to happen, only sleeps for 30 minutes and is awake again. There isn't always a solution, as napping well is a developmental work-in-progress and a real challenge too.

Under six months of age, I encourage you to follow the sleep-shaping guide as set out (see pages 60–3), building the loving-trust bond to lay a foundation for your baby's sleep. During the first six months you may find that you just need to help your baby day and/ or night sleep in any way that works. This may mean holding them in your arms, bouncing them on a yoga ball, rolling them in their pram, either in your home or out for a walk, wearing baby, and essentially doing your best to observe the suggested timings for their age and attempt to capture their sleep tendency *before* they become overtired – even if that means you are hugely involved in making this happen.

You will see from my suggestions in Chapter 5 that if you can work on the percentage-of-wakefulness approach at bedtime then you can see if you can phase this into the daytime for nap 1 or nap 2. But many parents just can't help their baby to go to sleep with ease or stay asleep for long and this may just be where your baby is at right now.

Lucy Says

I know it is really hard, but if you concentrate on helping them go to sleep and worry less about amounts of sleep you will probably be much better off emotionally and mentally too.

Certainly, the following adjustments can help to unlock naps, but often it will take until they're six months and over, together with a sleep-learning exercise, before your efforts can reasonably start to produce naps happening with relative ease and for long enough.

But I encourage you to observe the suggestions in the relevant chapters for this age range, along with the following:

- ☑ Always start the day no later than 7.30 a.m. (avoid starting the day before 6 a.m. – if your baby is alert after that, then get up and press start on the day).
- ☑ Expose your baby to bright natural light during wake times.
- ☑ Provide the first feed of the day outside of the bedroom so it does not feel like an extension of night-time.
- ☑ Acknowledge early sleep cues and act on them swiftly. If

you don't see sleep cues early in the morning, it is likely that baby needs to nap within 45 minutes to an hour and a half of getting up. This may seem like a small wake period for someone who has just risen, but this is the natural dynamic and it's useful to tie into it.

☑ If baby is willing, attempt the nap in the sleeper or cot – always do a pre-sleep ritual so they understand that it is time to sleep.

☑ From eight weeks onwards make the space for the nap dark – whether that is in a bedroom or the living space – to encourage sleep and to maintain it if possible.

☑ Use motion as needed to enable a nap, either at the start or mid-cycle.

☑ Don't worry about duration – naps at this age are very variable, ranging from 20 minutes to two to three hours, depending on the child. Don't spend any time trying to resettle them for a nap unless they are willing to go back to sleep or seem exhausted – again, maximum input from you is recommended.

☑ Wake your baby from naps to maintain your feeding practice as outlined.

☑ If you're making progress at bedtime with the percentage-of-wakefulness approach, then start nap 1 and nap 2 in the sleeper or cot.

☑ If you are not making progress, continue to address naps in any way that works and when ready, beyond six months, attempts naps in the cot with the stay-and-support approach as part of your sleep-learning exercise – don't waste your maternity leave trying for something that is not there to be had.

☑ Make sure that as your baby gets older you bring forward bedtime so that by four months it is around 7 p.m. – this can help initiate nap ability when it is ready to emerge.

☑ Avoid using the stay-and-support approach before six

months of age, as your baby may not be developmentally ready to learn that way.

Q Is timing really as important as you suggest?

Regardless of age, timing will always be the biggest barrier to achieving a nap. Observing early sleep cues and attempting a nap before your baby becomes overtired can actually make all the difference and, in some cases, transform the naps from 30-minute snapshots to an hour and more in duration.

As your baby gets older, having an age-relevant bedtime supported by my bedtime number line in association with the nap-gap dynamic and addressing the nap before your child becomes overtired is key.

> 'Pre-book-implementation we had inconsistent naps, anything from 20 minutes to three hours, and a bedtime that took one to two hours due to recurrent waking. Post-book we have consistent naps, three to four per day, lasting 40 minutes to two hours, and a bedtime that takes 10 minutes with low support and sleeping well until 7 a.m. Amazing – definitely picking up tiredness cues early is key! Looking forward to implementing your routine as he grows – honestly amazing!'
>
> – Vanessa, mum to 12-week-old Hugo

Amount of sleep

Q How much daytime sleep does my child need?

I try not to put too much emphasis on amounts of sleep or how many cycles of sleep your baby can get through. Of course they have a day-sleep need, but this can be achieved in a variety of ways and I find that parents are often chasing an elusive nap duration that most children cannot achieve.

Below is a guide, but it is just that: an idea of how much sleep is needed, which can vary from child to child. Mood and behaviour are good indicators of whether your baby is napping enough, and if naps are short then it may be a case of providing a series of short naps throughout the day – this often means that you don't get anything else done, but this may just be your journey and is why drafting in support is necessary, especially at the start. Better sleep ability emerges as your child gets older, and if in the first six months you don't get a result, then you can make further changes beyond six months to improve all your sleep segments, as discussed.

DAYTIME SLEEP NEEDS GUIDE

Age	Amount in hours	Number of naps	Comment
Up to 2 months	14–17 per 24	5–8 (possibly more)	Sleep is not organised Duration can be anything from 20 minutes to 2–3 hours
2–4 months	4–5	3–6	Sleep is not organised Duration can be anything from 20 minutes to 2–3 hours
4–6 months	3–4	3–5	Possibly getting more organised Duration from 30 minutes to 1–2 hours
6–8 months	3–3½	3–4	Naps possibly maturing Duration from 40 minutes to 1 hour+
8–12 months	2½–3	2–3	Higher chance of longer naps Duration from 40 minutes to 1 hour+
12–18 months	2 ¼–2½	1–2	Expect at least one nap Duration of 1 hour+

18–3 years	1–2+	1	Expect one nap Duration of at least 1 hour+
3 years+	0–2	0–1	Many no longer napping by 3 years Determined by individual child's needs

Q *My 10-month-old can already go to sleep at bedtime but is rocked to sleep for naps. When I try to help him nap in the cot he goes wild – any tips?*

From six months to about two years, you can generally successfully help your child to achieve their daytime sleep in the cot, if that is what you would like. Many parents rock or roll for daytime sleep, and if that works for you then no action is required. If, however, it is something you want to address then I encourage you to work on it. Also, if your child will attend daycare then it is best if the skill to sleep well in a cot is established at home and then transferred to daycare. Often we do this at the same time – we begin a sleep plan on the weekend and on the following Monday or so we look for the same approach in daycare.

For napping at home in the cot to become a possibility, you will need to either also begin to work on bedtime or be certain that your child has a complete (or in-progress) sleep ability at bedtime. This means no drinks of anything (even a sip of water) too close to bedtime, as this can lock out the nap ability. It will also be necessary to apply the age-relevant feeding and sleeping balance, as well as the fixed feed, the nap-gap dynamic and the bedtime number line. Ignoring this may mean your efforts to establish day sleep do not work.

Lucy Says

If you are beginning a whole plan, start at bedtime and the next day begin naps in the cot with the same approach. If it is just the naps you are working on, then start when you have a few days in a row to attempt it. But remember, you will need to be 100 per cent certain that the sleep ability at bedtime is already present or you will need to make changes at bedtime too for this to work. Your child also needs to be at least six months old or it may become an exercise in frustration for all.

Nap preparation

Q *I am worried about my baby crying for the nap, and then only sleeping for a short time*

Factors that cause crying at naptime:
- Under- or overtired
- Inadequate naptime routine
- Inadequate ability – either for naptime alone or for bedtime too – and thus needs to learn a new way to improve this, with your support

Factors that cause short nap durations:
- Timing – under- or overtired when nap is addressed
- Too much input at naptime stops the cycle from one sleep phase to another
- Inadequate environment

Nap preparation to help you overcome upset and improve nap location and ability:
- The nap must be timed as set out for your child's age range.
- The room *must* be dark – super-dark, even more so than at bedtime.
- You will need to provide a naptime routine as at bedtime – in the bedroom for *at least* 10 minutes, more if necessary. It may help if you go to the room 20 minutes before the end of the suggested wake period. This means if the wake period is two hours, that you take your baby to the room one hour and 40 minutes after getting up; if the wake period is three hours,

then take them two hours and 40 minutes after getting up or waking from the last nap.

- Pre-sleep ritual: dim the lights, close the curtains, change the nappy, put them into their sleeping bag; have song-time, story-time, lots of physical and eye contact. Get your baby nice and relaxed, or as relaxed as they can be, in the bedroom that they will nap in.
- Place your child in the cot – turn off music or white noise unless you plan to use it on a loop for the duration of the sleep period. It is essential that it does not switch off after sleep has been achieved.
- Once they're in the cot, sit beside them on the floor or a chair, depending on the level of the cot they are at – use all the strategies outlined in the stay-and-support approach (see page 26).
- Try for one hour to help your child take the nap. If after an hour they have not gone to sleep, then abort the mission – take them up and out of the room and have a change of scenery – but try again within the hour. If your first attempt does not work, don't to go back to your usual tactics such as feeding or rocking in your arms, or put them back in the buggy or car without first trying one more time in the cot.
- If the first attempt does not work, then do try again after about an hour. This may mean that your child is overtired, but that is OK for learning. It may also mean that your feed schedule is knocked out of sync, so adjust the next feed forward to avoid it clashing with this attempt. The day will be higgledy-piggledy, but don't worry about that – focus on mastering the ability at the onset of the nap.
- If the first attempt doesn't work then the second attempt generally will, and even if this nap is short – which is likely – the ability to go to sleep for the nap is starting to grow and the next day will hopefully be easier.
- The most likely dynamic is that the first attempt *will* work but your baby will wake up quite soon from the nap. Don't

worry about duration (I don't), only focus on application, so however long they sleep, unless they're really easy to resettle, get up, move on with the day, follow the wake period for the next nap and repeat.

- Only attempt a nap in the cot on two occasions in one day – either one nap that didn't work and one that did, two that worked but were short or two that didn't work. We won't go to the cot again that day, but if it is top heavy and nap sleep is over too soon, then provide a back-up or filler nap in the car or buggy, but without nursing or bottles or rocking – you could use the sling but the car or buggy would be preferable. Limit this nap as per your child's age range and stage; follow the bedtime number line and nap-gap dynamic, and bring forward bedtime as necessary to preserve the bedtime process and stabilise the night-time.
- Don't worry about the amount or duration of day sleep – that will emerge over the next three to four weeks as you work through the stages, or you may have to work on the mid-nap cycle as outlined below.

Nap imbalances

Q *I have started to help my child sleep in the cot, but he won't stay asleep – in the buggy he will nap for much longer*

When you begin to help your child to sleep in the cot for day sleep, the learning grows first at the going-asleep stage – it takes time for the longer sleep duration in the new location to emerge. It is also possible that, if you are working on all sleep segments, as your night-time sleep improves your daytime sleep-duration need is shrinking in response. Ultimately, you will establish your child's individual day-sleep need together with an optimised night-time sleep need.

Parents often talk about their child *only* sleeping for one sleep cycle (about 40 minutes), but I would encourage you to expect typically one nap of at least 40 minutes per day and another of at least an hour in duration. The two-hour nap is a rarity – of course it happens, but most children tend to sleep for 40 minutes to an hour and a half at a time. When your child is having a series of naps, then we try to have nap 2 as the stronger one – although nap 1 often wants to have that role.

Helping your child to sleep longer for a nap can emerge naturally as you work on the pieces of the puzzle, so for at least the first 10 days, just work on getting them to sleep – when that becomes an easier exercise we can turn our focus to keeping them asleep if necessary.

Lucy Says

Typically, nap 1 becomes easier to deliver quite quickly, so that within maybe a week of starting it's easily achieved and you can begin to move through the stages to sleep as outlined. Nap 2, if applicable, is a much trickier customer and may take two to three weeks to establish with lots of encouragement, as I will outline. But first let's master falling asleep and then we can look at staying asleep for the naps.

Allow the first 7–10 days to go by and then assess the situation. It is very likely than one nap is already getting longer – some parents report a doubling in length – while some of you will still be stuck with shorter naps.

If either nap 1 or nap 2 is under 45 minutes long, then try to resettle using stage 1 of the stay-and-support approach. Try this for at least 30 minutes and for seven days in a row before evaluating its efficacy.

It's important that the room is super-dark. It is also important that you are actively addressing any overnight activity because that can cause short naps. You must also be following the feeding layout and not feeding as soon as your child wakes from the short nap, which potentially ingrains the activity. It is also important that when they get up they are not carried in your arms all the time, as this may also be a reason for waking early.

After seven days, hopefully, you should see one or a combination of the following dynamics:

1. Your child starts to return to sleep with your input mid-nap – even if it's only for 10 minutes this is progress, and in time that will start to extend.

2. Sometimes, although you try, they never resettle, but after a few days the nap starts to lengthen – so the effort provided the yield just not in the moment.

If after seven days there is zero success – no longer naps and no instance where your child returned to sleep – then you may need to stop for a while, accept the length they are doing and continue to apply all the other measures, including moving the naps into place, as outlined in the next question.

Q *My day is top heavy – my child wakes early, naps early and short, and day sleep is finished too soon. The dilemma of early bedtime or too long a gap before bedtime seems to be causing a problem too.*

In the timing suggestions I outline in Chapter 9, there are two phases: wake-window-related timing and clock-based timing. I call moving to clock-based timing calibrating the day and you do this after ten days or so, provided nap one is getting easier to achieve in the cot, or wherever you have decided to nap your child. It doesn't need to be longer in duration yet – you can work on that as above – but now start to move your naps into position so that nap 1 (if applicable) is starting at 9 a.m. or beyond, despite the wake time, nap 2 has been adjusted as per your child's age range and the nap-gap dynamic is being observed too. This way we know that all your sleep stars are aligned to allow better, more rested and longer sleep tendencies if and when possible.

Transitions

🅠 I am unsure how to transition my child through their naps – from three naps to two, and two naps to one and so on …

Some nap transitions happen naturally and some need input from you – as with most things sleep, knowledge is power. Your baby will go through so many nap transitions in the first 18 months – from what feels like a million naps a day to a single one by 15–18 months!

At six to eight months, we see three to four naps per day, ideally, with one to two at least 40–45 minutes long, as well as one nap, ideally the second one, of at least an hour. I always wake after an hour and half for nap 1 to make sure there is enough room for nap 2. If in time there is only one long nap tendency, I will cut nap 1 to one hour to lengthen and strengthen nap 2 – this is the nap we prioritise, as it carries the can until bedtime and remains until closer to age three. Transitioning from three to four naps is quite natural – your child will start to be able to stay awake longer as the day unfolds, and as you calibrate the day you will slowly retire the extra naps, leaving you with two naps by eight months plus and a three- to four-hour wake period before bedtime.

Between 8 and 15 months we will generally see two naps per day – one nap of, ideally, at least 40–45 minutes and one of at least an hour. At this stage, while on two naps per day, each nap could be of equal duration, but if your child appears only able to have one long nap, then aim for this to be nap 2 by potentially waking on nap 1 after an hour or 45 minutes, depending, to allow this to happen. Strengthening nap 2 can help avoid being overtired at bedtime and reduce the risk of unnecessary night waking and early rising.

The 15–18 month age range is tricky, as we start to see a final transition from two daytime sleeps to one. It's important not to rush this transition and to only make it if you are seeing indications of the end of two naps – this is typically refusing either nap 1 or 2. Generally, if your child is this age and routinely visibly tired by 10 a.m. each day then they still need two naps – but you may have to limit nap 1 to

20–45 minutes, depending, for a second nap to be achievable. Again, ideally nap 2 is at least an hour but also finishing as close to 3–3.30 p.m. as possible so the nap-gap dynamic is observed, preserving your overall sleep goals.

For 18 months–2½ years one nap is generally appropriate, ranging from at least one to two hours per day. The retained nap is the original nap 2, and it is important that this nap happens close to 1 p.m. – even though sometimes your child may seem tired sooner – to observe the best balance for sleep pressure that enables more restful night-time sleep. So it should start at around 1 p.m. and finish as close to 2–3 p.m. as possible, observing the nap-gap dynamic.

Finally, somewhere from two-and-a-half to three years your child will start to drop their day sleep. When your child makes this final transition to no naps, they may either start to sleep less by day – 45 minutes to an hour and a half – or they may just start to skip days. It can take some time for your child to cope without daytime sleep, and bringing forward bedtime to 6–7 p.m. can help to offset a cycle of overtiredness and reduce the risk of night-time activity during this important transition.

Without a nap, providing quiet time around the time the nap would have routinely been offered is also a good solution, allowing your child to 'rest'. Lying on the couch and reading or listening to audiobooks can help them take a break from the busyness of days when they no longer need a sleep.

Daycare

Q *My child is in crèche and won't nap as long there as he does at home, meaning he is really tired when I collect him. This is leading to problems at bedtime and overnight.*

Napping in daycare can be a challenge – some children sleep less well and others much better than at home. As with most sleep issues, the sleep segments need to be addressed at home before we can expect adequate sleep durations in a strange environment – be that a crèche or a childminder's home. If you routinely support the naps at home in a way that your daycare won't be able to, such as nursing or rocking, then working on that may be necessary to improve day sleep in the crèche. The higher the level of sleep ability your child has at home, the greater the chance of their sleeping well in daycare. Working on the night-time sleep segment, if necessary, will mean that when your child is better rested by night they will likely sleep better by day, both at home and elsewhere.

It is helpful to supply your daytime layout to your daycare and get their positive input, especially if you are beginning a sleep-learning exercise. It is also useful to send familiar items from home to further support efforts to help your child sleep well there. One of the biggest barriers is that daycares routinely offer the main nap too early in the day, resulting in a long wake period before you can provide bedtime. Looking to move the naps later will take cooperation from *everyone* who is looking after your child. In my practice about 80 per cent of the children are in some form of daycare, and once the sleep issues are adequately addressed at home they tend to be transferable, but positive input is generally necessary until your child is better rested – then flexibility can be invoked.

Lucy Says

I could write a book on napping alone, as there are so many issues that parents experience and so many items to juggle to ensure your child is optimally rested. Of course, the controlling influences still tend to be bedtime and overnight, so don't disregard their significance when you attempt to resolve the issues you experience. One question I do see a lot is, if a child is doing things differently to how I propose, should it be changed? My reply will always be that as long as things are working for you, continue with no action – it is only when you want to make changes that you would start to make the adjustments I have outlined.

Chapter 15

Experts

C hildhood development is not one-dimensional, and each part of the puzzle has its own tendencies – sleep, breastfeeding, weaning, underlying medical issues – that contribute to your child's wellbeing. Each item exists independently but is co-dependent too. In my practice, I defer to experts in particular fields who I feel complement my work and can further support parents. In this chapter, I asked contributors to common questions that arise in their practice and hope that this will further help you on your journey.

Frank Kelleher, Paediatric Osteopath R.M.N.H., D.O., G.Os.C., O.C.I.

Frank has been working in healthcare for more than 30 years. His osteopathy journey began in 1992. He trained at the London School of Osteopathy and qualified in 1997. He returned to Cork in 1998 with his wife, Rose, and their family and set up his own clinic. Since then he has specialised in paediatric care and has built up a very busy practice. He has a far-reaching reputation, with parents travelling from all over Ireland to see him. One of Frank's main objectives is to give parents as much information as possible about their child's health. He is passionate about providing parents with an effective plan to help them manage and resolve the condition affecting their little one.

Q *My toddler got a few ear infections earlier this year and since then his sleep has deteriorated. Can paediatric osteopathy help?*

Ear infections are the most common illness to affect preschool children, with up to 90 per cent of children experiencing one before their third birthday. When an ear infection occurs, it is the middle ear that is affected. Some children just get the occasional ear infection, but others get recurring ear infections and it's generally these children we see at the clinic. They may also go on to develop glue ear as a result of fluid building up in the middle ear.

The middle ear is normally filled with air and is connected to the back of the nasal passages by a small tube called the Eustachian tube. This tube is short, narrow and horizontal in babies and toddlers and therefore not so effective. As a child grows the tube becomes more oblique and this allows fluid to drain from the middle ear much more effectively. This explains why some parents are often told that their child will 'grow out' of ear infections.

Children are frequently brought to see us because they don't sleep. On closer examination, we sometimes find that the child has had a few ear infections. In many cases like this, the child wakes at night because of the fluid in the middle ear. It may be uncomfortable, and the ears may need to pop. A little drink of water may help when they wake up, but the main aim of paediatric osteopathy treatment is to move the fluid and mucus away from the middle ear, relieving the pressure behind the eardrum.

Q *My son has a constant runny nose. He has never been a good sleeper. Are these connected?*

For children who have persistent colds and coughs, nasal drip could be an issue and a cause of sleep disruption. Children who have a nasal drip affecting the respiratory passages are often congested and frequently have a runny nose. They can be mouth breathers and as a result snore at night. This too can disrupt their sleep and wake them up. The other type of nasal drip is a posterior nasal drip, which, in this case, affects the back of the throat and the Eustachian tubes connecting the middle ear to the back of the throat, causing a cough and congestion. There can be nasal congestion too. These symptoms can disrupt the child's sleep. A product we recommend for children with nasal congestion is a salt pump. Used at night in the room the child sleeps in, it can help clear out the mucus and aid a good night's sleep.

Paediatric osteopathy treatment focuses on the cranial base using gentle techniques to enhance mucous drainage. Treatment opens up the ribcage motion by releasing intercostal muscle tension. This establishes a deeper breathing pattern and aids the movement of mucus in the respiratory system.

Q *Our daughter has had so many issues with reflux and allergy. How can I help her sleep?*

A common reason for sleep disruption is a digestive disorder. Reflux, wind or allergy can cause enough discomfort at night to wake a baby. They can be quite unsettled and tend to wake frequently. It's so important to manage the digestive disorder effectively. With reflux, for example, many babies can be very distressed at night due to the production of extra stomach acid between 2 a.m. and 5 a.m. If your baby is on medication and is unsettled at night, it's a good idea to give one of the late doses the first time they wake up after midnight. We see babies who are well and have been sleeping through the night for up to six or seven months. They then become unsettled and their sleep is affected. Some of these babies can have a mild sensitivity to cow's milk protein and it is only after they are weaned onto solids that it presents. Again, paediatric osteopathy can offer relief, along with specific advice depending on which condition is affecting baby. Once any cranial and physical issues are dealt with, baby should be able to develop a better sleeping pattern with a little help from their parents.

Q *My three-year-old daughter is waking a few times a week with night terrors. It's so stressful for us all. Can paediatric osteopathy help?*

Children often wake up upset after a bad dream or nightmare. In most cases, they can be settled and soothed and will go off back to sleep. With night terrors it's very different. 'Night terror' is a big term for what is essentially a type of bad dream. The child will cry out and be visibly distressed but is still sound asleep! They may shout for you but can't sense your presence or be comforted by you, making it difficult for you to soothe and reassure them. They will return to sleep after a period of 1–30 minutes but will not usually remember the details in the morning (although you will!).

While nightmares occur from dream sleep (rapid eye movement or REM sleep), night terrors occur from a deep non-dream sleep. A child may be able to recall a nightmare if they wake up but a child experiencing a night terror is not fully awake and will not remember the event.

Night terrors are common in children between the ages of three and eight years. The episode usually happens early in the night and they are more common in children with a family history of night terrors or sleepwalking.

Night terrors in a child are probably more distressing for the parents than they are for the child. They can occur after a traumatic event like a fall or a hospital admission, because of a change of schedule, a new baby in the house or stress or anxiety about something in their life, or if they are overtired and fall into a very deep sleep very quickly.

Night terrors will settle in time with reassurance but because they can be so distressing, many parents will look for a solution. Paediatric osteopathy is a very gentle treatment that works on the child's nervous system and breathing diaphragm and can be an effective way to treat them successfully.

Orla Dorgan, RGN Lactation Consultant

Orla is a practice nurse (RGN) working in a busy GP medical centre and is an International Board Certified Lactation Consultant (IBCLC). She is a mother to three young children. Orla has many years' experience helping many families with their newborns. She has a passion for helping families to establish breastfeeding and resolve any issues that may arise. She teaches introduction to breastfeeding classes for antenatal couples, empowering them with knowledge and giving them confidence. She also visits parents in their own home if they are experiencing breastfeeding difficulties and listens to their concerns, observing and helping to form a plan that will work for the family and help resolve any issues. Orla can be contacted on her website www.lactationtalk.com and is active on social media.

Q *What is a lactation consultant?*

An IBCLC provides breastfeeding support and evidence-based research to mums and their partners antenatally and postnatally.

Q *How do I know my baby is getting enough milk?*

Most babies lose 7 per cent of their birth weight after they are born. At 10 days old, we would expect the baby to have regained their birth weight. This is normal.

Other signs baby is getting enough milk are:

- 'Happy nappies' – plenty of dirty nappies, three to five in 24 hours
- Plenty of pale yellow or clear urine nappies, four to seven in 24 hours
- Being content and satisfied after a feed
- Switching happily between short sleeping periods and wakeful alert periods

Q How do I know when my baby is hungry?

You will see your baby starting to move. They may move their head from side to side, bring their hand to their mouth, make sucking noises. This is the best time to bring baby to the breast, when they are nice and calm. A calm baby will latch better than a baby at a late feeding cue, which is crying. You should not wait until your baby cries to feed them.

Q How do I know when my baby is full?

They may fall asleep at the breast. Their hands will splay out and be nice and relaxed. They will be content after the feed. They should sleep for short periods in between feeds. If your baby is having 8–12 feeds in a 24-hour period and they sleep in between, this is a great sign they are receiving enough milk per feed.

Q How long should I breastfeed for?

An average breastfeeding session can be anything from 20–40 minutes in the early weeks. Babies become more efficient as they get older and this time will lessen. Babies who feed for long periods at the breast may be not getting enough milk at a time. Cluster-feeding happens in the early weeks – this is where your baby can feed regularly over a two- to three-hour period in a day, often at evening time. They can be fussy during this time and this is normal. It lasts for only a few weeks.

Q What do I do if I have pain when breastfeeding?

Breastfeeding should not be painful except for mild tenderness in the early weeks at the start of a feed. Assess your latch and positioning. Get back to basics. Change positions. And don't delay in seeking help. Contact a local breastfeeding support group, public health nurse, GP/practice nurse, hospital IBCLC or a private lactation consultant. Getting to the root of the problem can save your breastfeeding journey.

Q What do I do if my baby refuses a bottle?

Don't panic! Most babies will refuse a bottle at some stage. This doesn't mean they will never take a bottle. But it can be stressful in the moment. Developmental milestones are a classic time when babies can be fussy and refuse the bottle. A good time to introduce a bottle can be when the baby is four weeks or older. You can use expressed breastmilk, as they are familiar with the taste. This gets your baby used to a new skill early. This is not to say they will not refuse a bottle later. If they are refusing a bottle, you can offer milk in a small cup (e.g. a medicine cup). It can be a bit messy but baby is receiving the milk. Let them play with an empty bottle, if they are old enough to hold one. This gets them familiar with the bottle and they won't be frightened of it. Play games with it, like pull and tug. Make it fun. When your baby is ready, they will bring the nipple of the bottle to their mouth. It's never a good idea to force a bottle into a baby's mouth as they could develop a permanent aversion to it. When your baby does start to take the bottle, ensure you practise paced bottle-feeding, so the flow of milk is nice and steady and they are not gulping. Some babies can be frightened by the fast milk flow so avoid gulping.

Q What can parents expect to achieve when they seek my support?

My passion is helping new mums, partners and their babies to breastfeed successfully. Empowering mum and dad before baby arrives gives them great confidence and can often lead to a successful breastfeeding journey. I offer holistic, honest and practical support to all parents. If they have taken my class and run into breastfeeding problems, they are a lot more confident and notice the problems at an early stage so they can be rectified early on. My classes are practical and all questions are answered in a relaxed environment, so you will learn everything you need to know.

I believe that every mother and baby deserves support during their breastfeeding journey. As an IBCLC, I am there to support breastfeeding families, especially if they encounter any difficulties. If it doesn't work out for these mums and baby, we lend a supportive ear and offer our help. Postnatally, I work with the mum, baby and partner in their own home. A full history is taken and observing baby at the breast is a big part of the consultation. Adjustments to breastfeeding positions to optimise comfort will be made and recommendations given for further care. We will draw up a plan together to help rectify the problem and get breastfeeding back on track. I follow up for two weeks afterwards to ensure breastfeeding is improving and mum and baby are reaching their breastfeeding goals. Support in these early weeks is crucial to a good breastfeeding journey and I believe every mum and baby deserves this.

Caroline O'Connor, Registered Dietitian and founder of Solid Start

Caroline is a registered dietitian, mum of four and founder of Solid Start. Solid Start offers parents no-nonsense evidence-based advice on food, feeding and nutrition for babies and young children. Caroline is registered with CORU and is a member of the Irish Nutrition and Dietetic Institute and a certified lactation consultant. Visit www.solidstart.ie for information on their classes and consultations.

Mounting scientific evidence shows that what we feed our babies really does matter. The first thousand days from birth to your baby's second birthday are a time of unprecedented growth and brain development, and proper nutrition is critical during this time. Weaning – the process of introducing solid foods alongside breast or formula milk – is a golden opportunity to lay down the foundations for lifelong health. What foods you choose to offer your baby and how you approach feeding in your family will influence their future health, food preferences and appetite regulation. So no pressure, parents!

In today's digital world there is no shortage of information available, but much of it is based on opinion or offered by people without appropriate qualifications. Given all the conflicting advice out there about what and how to feed babies, you may struggle to make sense of it all. Below are evidence-based answers to common questions about weaning and feeding babies. When it comes to information on food, feeding and nutrition, choose a registered dietitian for evidence-based advice you can trust.

Q Will starting solids improve my baby's sleep?

Parents are often advised by family and friends to start solids with the hope of encouraging their baby to sleep better at night. Unfortunately, there is no evidence that food and sleeping are linked. There are lots of reasons why babies wake at night that often have nothing to do with hunger. It is also possible they may be going through a growth spurt and need a little extra milk until they are ready to begin solids.

Q When should I start solids – I've been told four months by some and six months by others?

The age at which to start solids is one of the most debated topics on parenting forums and can be confusing when you receive conflicting advice.

However, the WHO and Irish and UK government guidelines all recommend waiting until around six months before starting solids. Waiting until six months is crucial because:

- Breastmilk is the best food for your baby during the first six months of life.
- Breastmilk or first infant formula provides all the energy and nutrients your baby needs until around six months, when they begin to need more iron and nutrients than breastmilk or formula alone can provide.
- At this age, your baby is developed enough to adequately cope with solid foods.
- Introducing foods at about six months (and not leaving it too long) helps your baby to develop essential skills such as self-feeding, and eating foods of different textures helps strengthen muscles that are important for later speech.

We say *around* six months because there is no perfect age and every baby is different. It's best to watch your baby for signs of readiness.

There are three clear signs that, when they occur together, show that your baby is ready for food. It is rare to see these three signs together before six months and never before four months.

The three vital signs your baby is ready for solids are:

- They can sit upright and hold their head up. This is important to ensure they can swallow food.
- They have good hand–eye coordination so they can look at food, pick it up and put it in their mouth.
- They can swallow food. If your baby is not ready, they will use their tongue to push the food back out of their mouth (this is known as the 'tongue thrust reflex').

Q How will I know when to reduce my baby's milk?

Breastmilk or first infant formula will continue to be your baby's main drink until twelve months of age, although you can use cow's milk in food at any time. Breastfed babies will naturally cut back on their feeds, maybe having shorter or less frequent feeds, when their food intake increases. On the other hand, some studies show that bottle-fed babies are more likely to continue drinking the same amount of milk while being introduced to solid foods. The average milk intake of a bottle-fed baby aged 7–9 months is approximately 600ml spread over three to four feeds and 400ml in babies aged 10–12 months spread over three feeds. Remember to be responsive to your baby and not encourage them to finish their milk if they are indicating they are full.

Q Which is better – baby-led weaning or spoon-feeding?

In years gone by, babies were weaned at a younger age onto runny purée fed to them from a spoon and at a much later stage were offered finger foods to eat themselves. In more recent times, baby-led weaning has become more popular. In baby-led weaning, babies feed themselves all their meals in the form of graspable pieces from day one – food is not given to the baby on a spoon at all. Today, Irish and UK guidelines recommend that babies are introduced to solids both by being offered small tastes of new foods on a spoon and by being given finger foods they can feed themselves. The reason is that there are pros and cons to self-feeding and spoon-feeding and both can be done well (they can also both be done poorly). So instead of choosing one approach over the other, why not take the best bits of baby-led weaning and spoon-feeding and combine them? This means keeping an open mind and realising that there are many different, but equally good, ways to feed a baby. As you'll find out when you start the weaning journey, what you want and what your baby prefers might be two different things!

Q What about baby fruit and vegetable pouches for the early days?

While prepared baby food is convenient, there are many reasons why preparing your own fruit and vegetables at home is better overall:

- Homemade fruits and vegetables have less free sugars. Commercial fruit and vegetable purées are high in free sugars, as sugar is released from the cell walls during high-speed blending and heat treating. Puréeing or mashing fruits and vegetables at home will not concentrate the sugars like this.
- The taste and colour will be authentic. Fruit and vegetable pouches lack the taste and colour of the real deal. Many, including those labelled as vegetables, are blended with fruit and sweeter vegetables. This makes it difficult for your baby to recognise the flavour, texture and appearance of individual fruits and vegetables and may reduce the likelihood that these will be accepted when served later as part of a family meal.
- The cost is much lower, and it's better for the environment.
- You can prepare a texture suited to your baby's stage. Pouches tend to be quite runny and many babies at six months are able for thicker purées or even mashed spoon feeds, as well as appropriate finger foods.
- Your baby can eat the same foods as the rest of the family and learn to recognise the smell, sight and taste of family foods rather than special 'baby foods' that they won't be eating later in life.

- Sucking food from a pouch does not teach the same eating skills as eating from a spoon or with your fingers.

Q What's the best food to start with?

Another hotly debated subject. You can start with any food you like! In some countries, iron-rich foods such as meat, eggs and fortified baby cereals are recommended as first foods. There is also some evidence to suggest that 'vegetable-first weaning' – a process whereby only single vegetables, notably harder-to-like green vegetables, are offered for the first one to two weeks – has benefits for the long-term acceptance of all vegetables.

Q How will I know how much food to offer?

There are no portion guidelines for babies. The golden rule is to feed your baby to appetite. It is up to you to schedule regular meals for your baby in addition to milk feeds. After this, it is up to your baby whether and how much of this food to eat. Start by offering minimal amounts – if your baby eats this and is eager for more, then offer more. The amount your baby eats will differ from meal to meal and day to day, and you'll soon recognise their needs:

- 'I'm hungry': I fuss, I'm excited, I reach for the spoon or food, I open my mouth, I lean towards you
- 'I'm full': I turn my head away, I spit food out, I push away the spoon or food, I close my mouth or cover it with my hands, I'm distracted, I fall asleep

Q Do I need to offer water with meals?

Yes, it's a good idea to introduce cooled, boiled water to babies with meals, regardless of whether you are breast or formula feeding. Using a small open cup is the best choice. Open-cup drinking requires sipping rather than sucking, which is like feeding from a bottle. Sipping is better for your baby's teeth. If you opt for a lidded beaker, choose one with a free-flowing spout rather than a non-spill valve, as these can lead to dental issues and even mouth development issues in the future.

Q Do I need to introduce foods one at a time?

No, this is not necessary for foods in general. However, potentially allergenic foods are best introduced one at a time in case of an allergic reaction. Ninety per cent of food allergies in children are caused by peanuts, tree nuts, fish, milk and eggs. These may be introduced at any time, and some evidence now supports adding these as early as you can. Babies at high risk of peanut allergy (those with severe eczema, egg allergy or both) should have peanut introduced following evaluation by an appropriately trained specialist.

Q I'm worried about choking – what foods are unsafe for my baby?

Choking is a common fear among new parents, particularly when thinking about introducing finger foods. However, the BLISS study in New Zealand showed that infants following a version of baby-led weaning, modified to reduce the risk of choking, did not appear to choke more often than infants weaned using a traditional approach. This suggests that baby-led approaches to weaning can be as safe as conventional spoon-feeding methods provided parents are given the appropriate safety advice. However, high proportions of infants in both groups were shown to be offered foods posing a choking risk, infants were not consistently closely supervised while eating and a small number of serious choking events were observed in both groups.

You should take the following precautions to keep your baby safe during weaning:

- Test finger foods to make sure they are soft enough to mash between two fingers (or are large and fibrous enough that small pieces do not break off when sucked and chewed, like a strip of steak).
- Avoid offering foods that form a crumb in the mouth.

- Make sure that the first finger foods are at least as long as your baby's fist.
- Make sure your baby is always sitting upright when eating.
- Always watch your baby while eating or playing with food.
- Never let anyone except your baby put whole foods into their mouth.
- Learn the difference between gagging and choking.
- Avoid foods known to be a choking risk such as raw vegetables, raw apple and hard underripe fruit, whole or chopped nuts, popcorn, round fruits (unless chopped), and food cut into coins, like sausages.
- Take a baby first-aid class.

Lucy Says

Caroline also very kindly answered some common questions in relation to reflux and cow's milk protein allergy, which comes up a lot in my practice. In order for sleep to start to get better, we generally need any digestive discomfort managed and controlled, but often it is hard to see what is causing what. Here's what Caroline has to say.

Q What is reflux?

Reflux is the medical term for 'spitting up'. It occurs when the contents of the stomach come back up into the oesophagus or mouth. It's also called gastro-oesophageal reflux, regurgitation, posseting or silent reflux (when the stomach contents don't make it all the way up and out of the mouth).

Q How common is reflux?

Reflux is a normal process that occurs in healthy babies, children and adults. When this happens to us as adults, we have the benefit of gravity, so all that tends to escape is gas in the form of a burp! But a baby is lying down much of the time so what escapes tends to be milk. Most babies have brief episodes during which they spit up milk through their mouth or nose. This does not usually bother them, does not lead to any complications and does not require treatment. Babies who spit up frequently but feed well, gain weight normally and are not unusually irritable are usually considered 'happy spitters'. Reflux is commonly blamed for irritability; however, excessive crying and reflux are both common conditions in babies and, therefore, they often coincide without being necessarily related.

Reflux usually begins before eight weeks of age. It may be frequent, with some babies having six or more episodes every day, typically peaks at four months and resolves in 90 per cent of babies by one year of age.

Q Why is reflux so common in babies?

Babies triple their body weight in the first year of life and therefore need lots of calories relative to their small size. This means that their tummy is often full, triggering the muscle at the top of the stomach to open, allowing the stomach contents to escape. It's the equivalent of us adults drinking a couple of litres of milk every three to four hours and then lying down in between!

Q When does reflux become a problem?

While reflux is normal, in a small number of babies, it may cause signs of distress or lead to certain complications that need medical management. This is known as gastro-oesophageal reflux disease (GORD). Some of the signs that your baby might have GORD include refusing to feed, frequently crying and arching the neck and back as if in pain, choking while spitting up, forceful or projectile vomiting, spitting up blood, frequent coughing or not gaining weight. Many of these symptoms, however, occur in babies with or without GORD. If excessive irritability and pain are the only symptoms, then it is unlikely to be related to GORD.

Q What are the best positions for your baby?

- Placing your baby in upright positions may help keep food in the stomach by gravity. When your baby's body is slumped, pressure on the tummy can push food out. Careful positioning keeps your baby's body upright and straight. If you see 'wrinkles' on your baby's tummy, it means that they are not upright.

- Swings and bouncy seats can work well to keep your baby upright. Use rolled blankets or towels to keep their body straight when they are slumping. Car seats cause babies to slump, which increases the pressure in the stomach and can make reflux worse.
- Tummy time in an elevated position at 30 degrees is beneficial, but this shouldn't be used for sleeping due to the risk of SIDS. Babies must be supervised in this position.
- If your baby shows signs of reflux during nappy changes, prop your baby on a low wedge or pillow. Roll your baby to the side to wipe their bum, rather than lifting both legs into the air. Try to time changes before feeding, when the stomach is most empty.
- Choose a front carrier that keeps your baby upright and straight – a lot of slings tend to 'bend' your baby.
- Holding your baby at your shoulder keeps them very upright and the body straight. Your baby can be comfortable on their back in your lap if your knees are bent enough to keep your baby upright.

FEEDING STRATEGIES THAT CAN HELP

- When breastfeeding, make sure your baby is at an angle and not flat. Laid-back breastfeeding positions can help with this. Speak with a certified lactation consultant to check that your baby is latched on well and to advise on managing high milk supply, a forceful letdown and tongue tie, as these can also impact on reflux.
- When bottle-feeding, be sure to hold your baby in a position with the body upright and straight and try paced bottle-feeding to avoid 'guzzling' of feeds. Use an anti-colic teat and make sure the hole is not too large. Avoid shaking the

feed when you're making it up as this traps air, which is then swallowed.

- Small, frequent feedings may help reduce reflux. Follow your baby's hunger signals but try to space feedings two to three hours apart. Your baby will take less and not overfill their stomach.
- When you burp your baby sitting on your lap, be sure their body is straight upright, not leaning forward or slumping.
- Keeping your baby upright and still for 15 to 30 minutes after feeding may help. When your baby's stomach is full, sudden movements and position changes may cause reflux.
- Thickening feeds or using pre-thickened formula may slightly improve visible regurgitation and vomiting in babies. But it is uncertain whether the use of food thickeners improves other signs and symptoms of reflux. Talk to a registered dietitian about thickening feeds or using specialised formula.

Q Reflux and cow's milk protein allergy

It is reported that up to 40 per cent of babies with GORD (not normal reflux) have a delayed cow's milk protein allergy. This should be appropriately diagnosed by a registered paediatric dietitian before cutting out cow's milk food in your own diet if you are breastfeeding or switching to a specialised formula if you are bottle-feeding.

Q Reflux medications

You will need to speak with your GP or paediatrician to discuss whether medications are necessary for your baby. Medicines called alginates (e.g. Gaviscon) can be used in the short term if the positioning and feeding tips above haven't been helpful. Acid-suppressing medications are only recommended for babies with an inflamed oesophagus caused by GORD and not for the treatment of crying and distress or for the treatment of visible regurgitation in otherwise healthy babies.

Appendix

Safe sleep to reduce the risk of SIDS

☑ Always place your baby on their back to sleep.
- Babies who sleep on their tummies have a higher risk of cot death.
- It is not safe to place your child on their side.
- When your baby is older and able to roll from back to front and back again, let them find their own sleep position, always having placed them on their back at the start of sleep.

☑ Keep your baby smoke-free before and after birth.
- Smoking greatly increases the risk of cot death.
- Don't allow anyone to smoke in the home or car.
- If either parent smokes, you should not share a bed with your baby.

☑ Carefully think through bed-sharing based on the recommendations. Bed-sharing can also increase the risk of suffocation or entrapment. Do not share a bed with baby if:
- either parent smokes (even if not in the home)
- either parent has taken alcohol, drugs or medication, or
- you are extremely tired.

OR

If your baby is:

- less than three months old
- was born prematurely (before 37 weeks), or
- had a low birth weight (less than 2.5kg or 5.5lbs).

☑ The safest place for baby to sleep is in a cot in your bedroom for at least 6 months.

- Place your baby with their feet to the foot of the cot so that they cannot get underneath the covers.
- Tuck covers in loosely and securely but not higher than baby's shoulders and ensure that they cannot slip over baby's head.
- Make sure your baby's head stays uncovered.
- Keep the cot free of loose and soft bedding, toys, bumpers, duvets, etc.
- Use a cot mattress that is clean, firm and flat and that fits the cot correctly. The mattress should be new for each child.

☑ Don't let baby get too hot.

- An overheated baby is at an increased risk of cot death.
- Don't wrap your baby in too many blankets.
- Cellular cotton blankets are best.
- Do not use duvets, quilts or pillows.
- Baby should not wear a hat.
- Ensure the room temperature is ranging from 16–20°C (62–68F).
- Never place the cot near a radiator, heater or fire, or in direct sunlight.

☑ Breastfeed your baby, if possible.

- Breastfeeding reduces the risk of cot death.
- Try to breastfeed for as long as you can.

☑ Consider a dummy.

- Some studies suggest that using a dummy each time your baby goes for a sleep reduces the risk of cot death.
- If you are using a dummy, then offer it at each sleep time.

- If you are breastfeeding, delay the introduction for a month until feeding is established.
- Don't worry if the dummy falls out when sleeping.
- Don't force the dummy if your baby is resistant.
- Don't attach the dummy with strings or cords.
- Never dip the dummy in sugar, syrup, honey or other food or drink.

☑ Provide tummy time with supervision. When your baby is awake, let them spend some time on their tummy and sitting up while you supervise.

- It is recommended to do this from birth.
- Always place baby on a firm, flat surface.
- Ideally, do this three times per day for 3–5 minutes and slowly build to longer sessions.

☑ Car seats, swings, infant seats and similar devices are not recommended for routine sleep in the house. Never fall asleep with your baby on the couch or armchair as the risk increases dramatically.

- Sleeping sitting up can cause problems with breathing.
- Once asleep, transfer your baby onto their back to sleep as soon as is practical.
- Babies should not be left unsupervised in a seated position for long periods of time.

If your baby seems unwell, get medical advice early and quickly. For more information, see sidsireland.ie.

INDEX